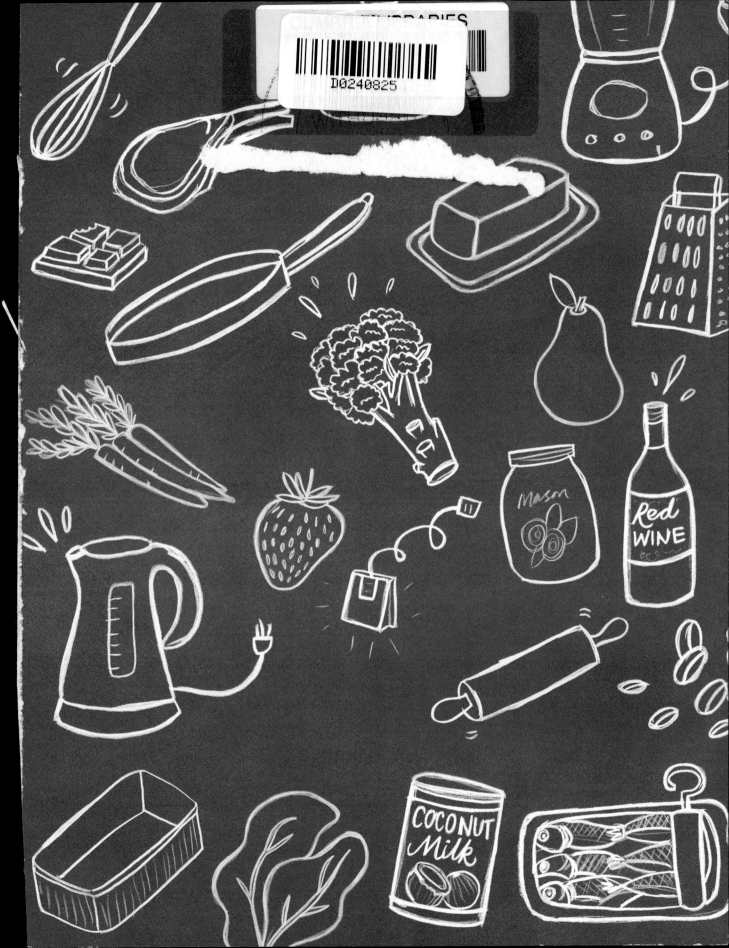

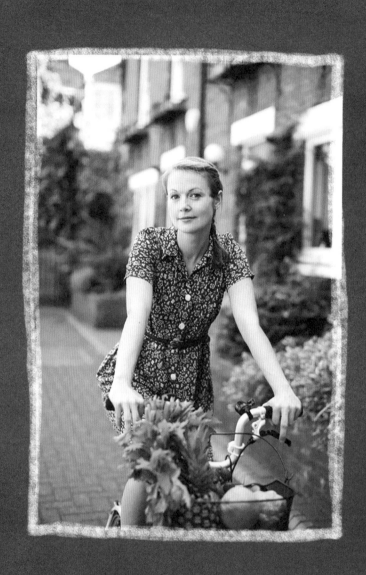

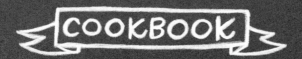

COOKBOOK

Irena Macri was born in Ukraine and moved to Australia
at the age of sixteen. She graduated from the College of
Fine Arts at UNSW with a Bachelor of Digital Media. In
2012 she founded the popular blog Eat Drink Paleo.

Irena is a digital nomad and an avid traveller.
She divides her time between London and Sydney.

MICHAEL JOSEPH

UK | USA | Canada | Ireland | Australia
India | New Zealand | South Africa

Michael Joseph is part of the Penguin Random House group of companies
whose addresses can be found at global.penguinrandomhouse.com.

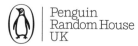

First published by Irena Macri, 2013
This edition published by Michael Joseph, 2015

001

Design by Carla Hackett
Photographs by Irena Macri
Edited by Jodie McLeod
Author photographs by Tony C French
Typeset in Archer and Verlag by Carla Hackett
Colour reproduction by TAG Publishing
Printed in Italy by Printer Trento SrL

A CIP catalogue record for this book is available at the British Library

ISBN 978-0-718-18165-9

www.greenpenguin.co.uk

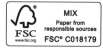
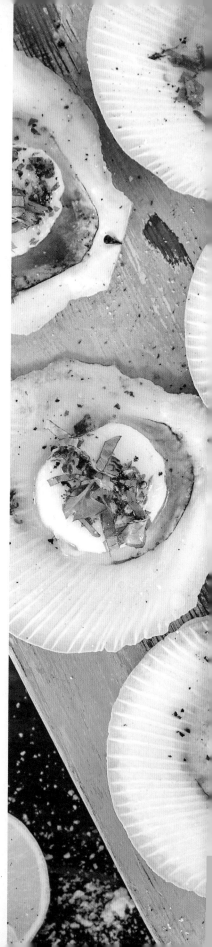

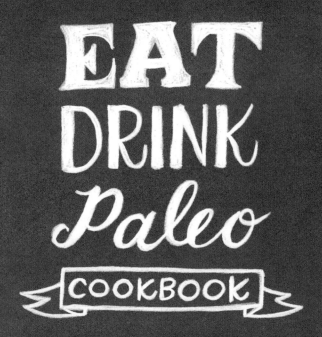

IRENA MACRI

MICHAEL JOSEPH
an imprint of
PENGUIN BOOKS

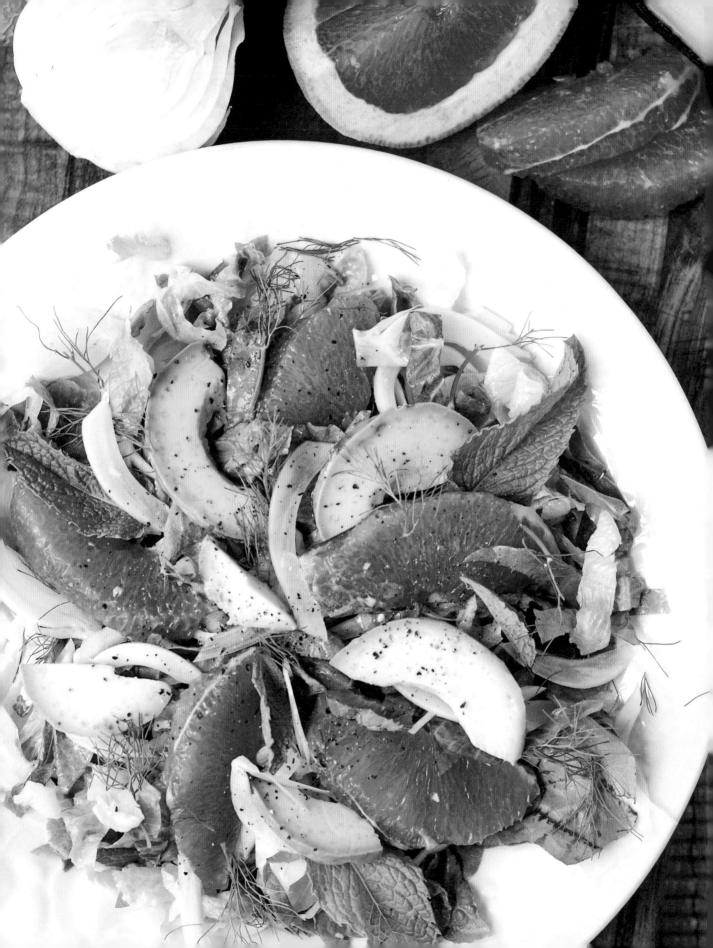

contents

Welcome

Thank you for purchasing my cookbook. The fact that you did means that you and I are very much alike – we enjoy good food, we care about our wellbeing, we love to cook and have fun in the kitchen, and outside. Perhaps you're not all of the above but I bet we could be friends. So let me introduce myself and tell you a little story of how this cookbook came to be.

my journey

It all started in May, 2012, when I quit my corporate job to pursue a passion – read: obsession – for cooking and all the other things that qualify me as a life-long foodie. Yes, I know, there are millions of other people who share the same passion – hello *MasterChef* and *Saturday Kitchen* – but I'm talking about a slightly different fixation. What I have, and I've had it ever since I cooked my first dish in my grandmother's kitchen, is an insatiable desire to play with food – to whisk it, mould it, whip it, sizzle it and drizzle it till the cows come home. For a long time now, I've seen the kitchen as a playground where I can create and let my instincts go wild, where I experiment and where I don't follow instructions. It's a feeling of wanting everyone else to see cooking through my eyes and to show that it's completely normal to get stupidly excited about a truffle mushroom or a piece of amazing grass-fed beef. And waking up in the middle of the night to write down a recipe I just dreamt about because I feel like it's the most brilliant one I've ever come up with and everyone will love it.

This 'inner vocation' slowly grew into a nebulous dream, but for a long time I didn't know what to do with it. I left it there like a reserve batter, sitting on a side bench of a playing field. I kept looking for an outlet, something to pour my passion for food into. I thought about going to a culinary school, opening my own wine bar or a café, starting a catering business and, yes, maybe for just one second, I imagined going on *MasterChef* or some other cooking contest. None of it sat well in my head or in my heart. I like to believe I'm a 'live in the moment, be free, make your own rules' kind of gal and I just couldn't commit.

Then I discovered paleo, a diet and lifestyle I will touch on in the next chapter, and everything fell into place. I found a way to combine my passion for cooking with my skills and background in digital media and create something that allowed me to play by my own rules. My website, Eat Drink Paleo, was born.

Focusing on paleo was a no-brainer for me – I was getting into the lifestyle and feeling fantastic as a result, and I was cooking a bunch of great, new food and trying new ingredients. At the same time there was a lack of exciting, paleo-friendly recipes around. It was a perfect combination – an opportunity to unleash my culinary experiments and kitchen prowess; to learn and, consequently, educate others on how to feel great by eating real, delicious food. In addition, I felt the need to demystify paleo as a diet, which I thought was perceived as a fad or as a boring, impractical, restrictive and meat-heavy way of eating. I knew first-hand that it doesn't have to be that way and that my approach – flexible, affirmative and personal – is an easier way to integrate the paleo diet into your life.

For nine months I've been developing, testing and photographing paleo-inspired recipes for the site, building a community, educating myself and advocating good nutrition and healthier lifestyle habits. My audience grew quickly and I knew I was on to something. You know you're doing something right when you start receiving emails and comments from real people telling you they had a fabulous dinner with their family thanks to your recipes, or that your content and passion inspires them on their journey. I realised that I'd found a way to connect.

Making a cookbook was a natural progression. I had so many fantastic recipes in my head and I really wanted to produce something that was different to what was available. I envisioned a cookbook that reflects my 80/20 philosophy, showcases real food and natural ingredients, and screams '*cooking is fun*'.

> ## My 80/20 philosophy
> ### screams 'cooking is fun!'

This cookbook is direct from the heart of someone who really loves to cook. It's been created in a very small kitchen using basic equipment and common ingredients, demonstrating that the recipes can be cooked by pretty much anyone. It's also special because it was originally self-published and made possible by many friends and strangers who believed in my crazy dream and gave me an unbelievable opportunity to share it with you.

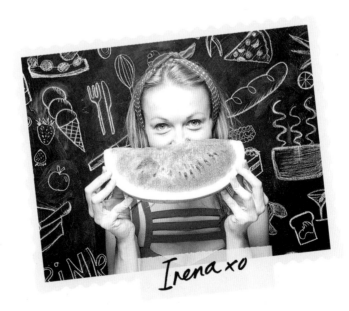

Irena xo

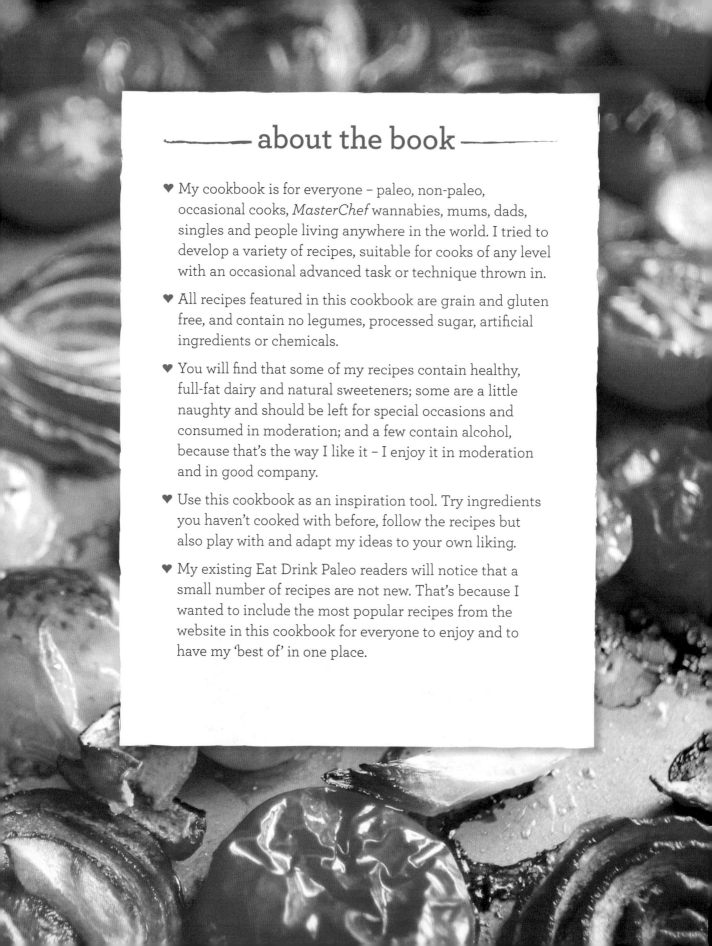

about the book

♥ My cookbook is for everyone – paleo, non-paleo, occasional cooks, *MasterChef* wannabies, mums, dads, singles and people living anywhere in the world. I tried to develop a variety of recipes, suitable for cooks of any level with an occasional advanced task or technique thrown in.

♥ All recipes featured in this cookbook are grain and gluten free, and contain no legumes, processed sugar, artificial ingredients or chemicals.

♥ You will find that some of my recipes contain healthy, full-fat dairy and natural sweeteners; some are a little naughty and should be left for special occasions and consumed in moderation; and a few contain alcohol, because that's the way I like it – I enjoy it in moderation and in good company.

♥ Use this cookbook as an inspiration tool. Try ingredients you haven't cooked with before, follow the recipes but also play with and adapt my ideas to your own liking.

♥ My existing Eat Drink Paleo readers will notice that a small number of recipes are not new. That's because I wanted to include the most popular recipes from the website in this cookbook for everyone to enjoy and to have my 'best of' in one place.

about me

- ♥ I was born in Ukraine, in a small city near the Carpathian Mountains. I moved to Australia when I was 16 years old.

- ♥ I had an unusually developed palate when I was a child – I was obsessed with salo, a type of Russian salty lard, loved herring, olives, salami and liver pate, and I even ate raw meat.

- ♥ Sydney, Australia, is my home but I'm a bit of a digital nomad. I love Tuscany in Italy for food, Tonsai in Thailand for adventure and Tokyo in Japan for all the craziness.

- ♥ I eat paleo 80 per cent of the time with the remaining 20 per cent consisting of occasional butter, cheese, rice, quinoa, fresh corn, beer, dumplings and gelato.

- ♥ I learnt to cook from my family, through my travels and by watching lots of cooking shows. I own a lot of cookbooks and food magazines but I hardly ever cook from recipes.

- ♥ My foodie icons include Jamie Oliver, Maggie Beer, Lotta Lundgren, Nigella Lawson, Heston Blumenthal and my inspiring late grandmother.

- ♥ My favourite ingredients are butter, garlic, lemon, olive oil, chilli, avocado, sweet potato, broccoli, gherkins, grass-fed beef, berries, coconut cream and anything with truffles.

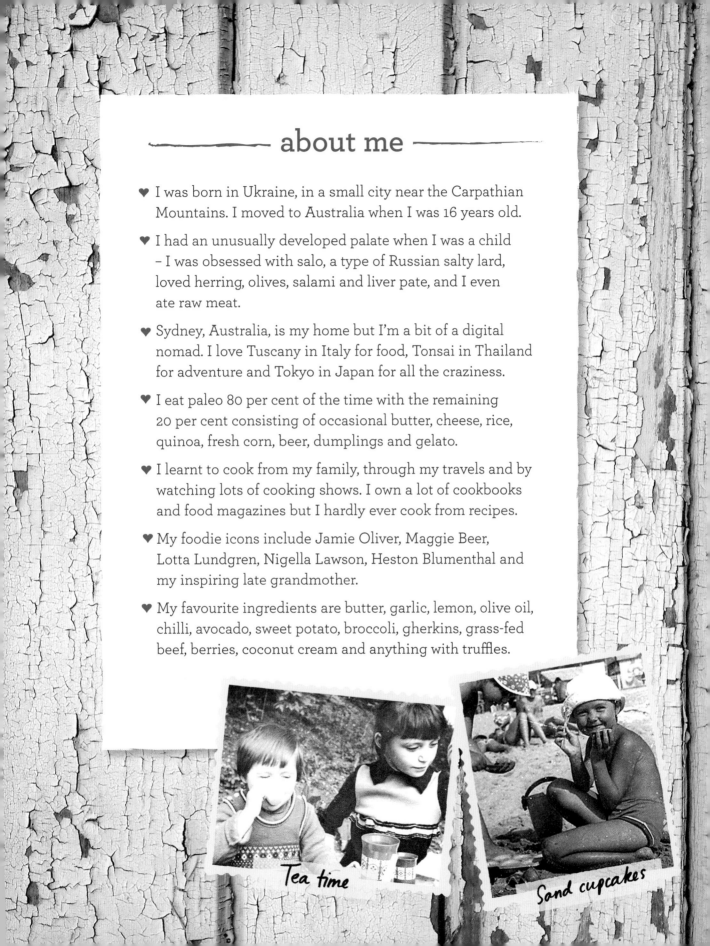

Tea time

Sand cupcakes

as you go along

Get familiar with these icons to help you navigate and filter through the recipes.

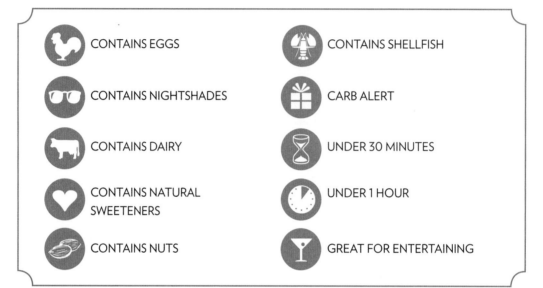

CONTAINS EGGS

CONTAINS SHELLFISH

CONTAINS NIGHTSHADES

CARB ALERT

CONTAINS DAIRY

UNDER 30 MINUTES

CONTAINS NATURAL SWEETENERS

UNDER 1 HOUR

CONTAINS NUTS

GREAT FOR ENTERTAINING

Recipes are divided into the following sections:

WAKE UP BABY
Delicious, satiating food ideas to kick-start your day.

FROM THE GARDEN
Salads, soups and sides made with vegetables, mushrooms, nuts, seeds and fruits.

MEAT
Recipes using a variety of meats as the key ingredient.

FISH 'N' FRIENDS
Fish, prawns, oysters and much more.

CHEEKY TREATS
Desserts and sweet treats for special occasions, weekends and entertaining.

QUICKIES
Snacks and small plates for parties and ideas for food on the go.

MAKE YOUR OWN
Make your own sauces, condiments, dips, stock and yoghurt.

BOTTOMS UP
Originals and paleo adaptations of the classic cocktails, shakes and smoothies.

paleo know-how

ROBB WOLF I owe a lot of my paleo know-how to this guy. A former research biochemist, Robb wrote the *New York Times* bestseller, *The Paleo Solution: The Original Human Diet*, which was the book that convinced me to try paleo. I'm a regular listener of his highly entertaining weekly podcast and I often visit his website when looking for nutrition and fitness information. I love his sensible approach and his sense of humour.

MARK SISSON The George Clooney of the paleo world, Mark is an American fitness author and blogger known for his book *The Primal Blueprint* and his highly informative website on all things primal, Mark's Daily Apple.

CHRIS KRESSER For more in-depth science behind the paleo framework and nutrition in general, check out Chris Kresser's website. His posts are lengthy, nerdy and contain just the right dose of healthy skepticism.

Astrophysicist and software entrepreneur **PAUL JAMINET, PH.D.** and his wife, **SHOU-CHING SHIH JAMINET, PH.D.**, a molecular biologist and cancer researcher, are the brains behind the *Perfect Health Diet* book and website. The geek in me loves the information they provide and the cook in me loves that they approve white rice and dairy foods.

CLAIRE YATES An Australian nutritional medicine practitioner and the founder of Indi Nature, a health and wellbeing blog, Claire is passionate about education and helping clients with digestive problems and emotional eating. Claire was one of the first practising paleo nutritionists in Australia and is registered with the global evolutionary healthcare group, Primal Docs. I was fortunate enough to collaborate with Claire on *Rejuvenate* – a health and wellbeing programme, which led to the creation of our joint website *Rejuvenated For Life*.

DIANE SANFILIPPO The founder of Balanced Bites and the author of *Practical Paleo*, Diane is another cool cat on the paleo streets. She is a sassy, classy and smart holistic nutritionist specialising in paleo nutrition, blood-sugar regulation, food allergies/intolerances and digestive health.

SALLY FALLON The co-founder of The Weston A. Price Foundation and author of *Nourishing Traditions*, a book every foodie and cook should read.

More resources and reading on the Eat Drink Paleo website.

Paleo Basics

This cookbook won't give you all the hows and whys of the paleo diet. I believe there are much better books and resources written by experienced evolutionary biologists, biochemists, nutritionists and doctors. However, for those of you completely new to paleo, here is what you need to know.

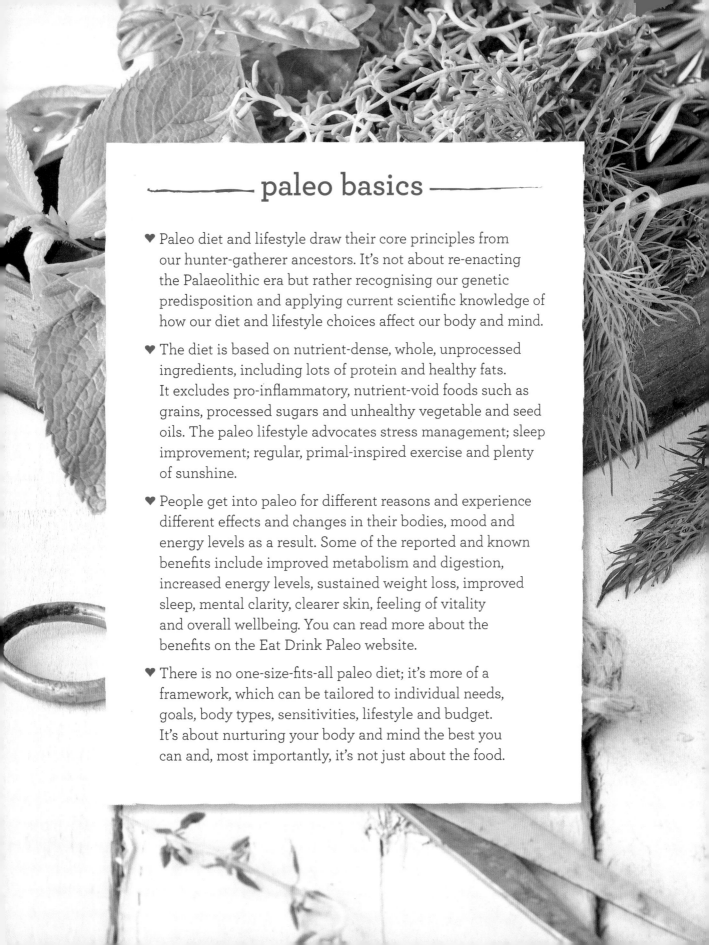

paleo basics

♥ Paleo diet and lifestyle draw their core principles from our hunter-gatherer ancestors. It's not about re-enacting the Palaeolithic era but rather recognising our genetic predisposition and applying current scientific knowledge of how our diet and lifestyle choices affect our body and mind.

♥ The diet is based on nutrient-dense, whole, unprocessed ingredients, including lots of protein and healthy fats. It excludes pro-inflammatory, nutrient-void foods such as grains, processed sugars and unhealthy vegetable and seed oils. The paleo lifestyle advocates stress management; sleep improvement; regular, primal-inspired exercise and plenty of sunshine.

♥ People get into paleo for different reasons and experience different effects and changes in their bodies, mood and energy levels as a result. Some of the reported and known benefits include improved metabolism and digestion, increased energy levels, sustained weight loss, improved sleep, mental clarity, clearer skin, feeling of vitality and overall wellbeing. You can read more about the benefits on the Eat Drink Paleo website.

♥ There is no one-size-fits-all paleo diet; it's more of a framework, which can be tailored to individual needs, goals, body types, sensitivities, lifestyle and budget. It's about nurturing your body and mind the best you can and, most importantly, it's not just about the food.

what's in

The following foods get a paleo seal of approval. Depending on the condition of your health, lifestyle and goals, some of these foods should be consumed in moderation. If you're trying to lose weight, improve your metabolism or if you're suffering from insulin resistance or autoimmune-related diseases, intake of vegetables and non-grain flours high in carbohydrates and fruit high in sugar should be kept to a minimum. Some people need to avoid eggs, dairy or nightshades, while others can enjoy them freely. Please consult your doctor or a qualified nutritionist on how to best adapt the paleo diet to your needs.

MEAT, SEAFOOD & EGGS

Beef, veal, lamb, kangaroo, pork, venison, game meats, bison, buffalo, goat, mutton, rabbit, chicken, duck, quail, pheasant, pigeon, goose, turkey, ostrich, emu, crocodile, and organ meats such as liver, kidneys and hearts. Chicken eggs, quail eggs.

Most fish, especially oily fish, prawns, shrimp, oysters, clams, mussels, snails, lobster, crab.

> ♥ *Eat meat from grass-fed animals, butter from grass-fed cows, and free-range poultry and eggs. It's more nutritious and better for the planet and the animals.*
>
> ♥ *When buying sausages, look for gluten-free varieties with natural ingredients and as few additives and preservatives as possible.*
>
> ♥ *If you can't find any grass-fed meat in your local supermarket, try ordering online or directly from the farm.*
>
> ♥ *When buying fish and seafood, look for the most sustainable varieties available. Oily fish, such as sardines, salmon and trout, are very high in omega-3 fatty acids and calcium, while shellfish is well known for its high content of minerals.*

WHAT ABOUT DELI MEATS?

If you're like me, you absolutely love cured meats – salami, prosciutto, bacon, chorizo and ham off the bone. Some paleo purists avoid cured meat but there isn't much harm in consuming good quality, naturally cured meats in moderation. Sure, they're salty, but we need some salt; and they might contain nitrate or nitrite but so do many other foods we eat; and, as Chris Kresser pointed out in his post on bacon, 'there is no reason to fear nitrates and nitrites in food', especially the amounts present in cured meats. Bring on the bacon!

VEGETABLES

Most of the carbohydrates in the paleo diet come from vegetables, tubers (stem and root vegetables) and fruits. Your personal carbohydrate needs depend on your health and lifestyle. Mark Sisson, author of *The Primal Blueprint*, recommends consuming between 100 and 150 grams of carbohydrates per day for effortless weight maintenance, between 50 and 100 grams for moderate fat loss and below 50 grams for accelerated fat loss. The intake can be higher for athletes and regular exercisers who need to replace post-workout glycogen stores.

Low carb (under 10 grams of carbohydrates per 100 grams)

Asparagus, aubergine, avocado, bamboo shoots, beet greens, bok choy, broccoli, brussels sprouts, bean sprouts, cabbage, cauliflower, cavolo nero, celery, chard, collard greens, courgette, courgette flowers, cucumbers, daikon radish, dandelion greens, endive, fennel, garlic, green beans, green onions, kale, kohlrabi, lettuce, mangetouts, mushrooms, mustard greens, okra, onion, peppers, pumpkin, radicchio, radishes, rhubarb, rocket, savoy cabbage, seaweed, shallots, spinach, spaghetti squash, swede, tomatillos, tomatoes, turnips, turnip greens, watercress.

Medium carb (10–20 grams of carbohydrates per 100 grams)

Artichokes, beetroot/beets, butternut squash, carrots, green peas, Jerusalem artichokes, leeks, lotus root, parsnips.

High carb (more than 20 grams of carbohydrates per 100 grams)

Cassava, taro, plantains, potato, sweet potatoes, winter squash, yams, yuccas.

♥ *Fresh is always best but frozen vegetables are still packed with nutrients and can be used freely if more convenient.*

♥ *Traditionally fermented vegetables are highly nutritious due to their probiotic properties.*

♥ *Depending on the ingredients and the preparation method, pickled vegetables can also retain most of their nutrients.*

♥ *Canned vegetables are usually pre-cooked and contain very little in nutrients by the time they get on your plate.*

♥ *When using potatoes specifically, make sure to peel them to remove some of the anti-nutrients found in the skin.*

FRUIT AND BERRIES

Low sugar (under 7 grams per 100 grams)

Avocado, blackberries, blueberries, blackcurrant, boysenberries, cranberries, gooseberries, grapefruit, green mango, green papaya, huckleberries, lemon, lime, mulberries, papaya, raspberries, redcurrant, salmon berries, star fruit, strawberries.

Medium sugar (7–15 grams per 100 grams)

Apples, apricots, cantaloupe melon, cherries, guava, honeydew melon, fresh figs, kiwi fruit, oranges, passionfruit, peaches, pears, persimmons, pomegranate, plums, tangerines.

High sugar (more 15 grams per 100 grams)

Bananas, grapes, lychees, mangos, nectarines, pineapple, plantains, watermelon.

FATS & OILS

The paleo diet embraces saturated fats and healthy plant-based oils and avoids highly refined and processed polyunsaturated oils, such as canola, vegetable oil and margarine, due to their toxic properties and high omega-6 fatty acids. Your fat intake should come from meat, seafood, eggs, nuts, avocados and fats and oils used in food preparation. It's important to know which type of fat or oil is best suited to which food preparation method.

♥ *Saturated fat is typically more heat stable and doesn't oxidate as quickly as monounsaturated and polyunsaturated fats, which makes it more suitable for frying and other high-temperature cooking.*

♥ *Nut oils and olive oil are more fragile and can be cooked with but are best used unheated to retain the most antioxidants, vitamins and flavour.*

♥ *Refined oils will usually have a higher smoking point. Ideally, they should be expeller-pressed, which indicates that the oil was extracted using a mechanical process rather than with heat and chemicals. These are best for high-temperature cooking such as deep-frying.*

OLIVE OIL

From highest to lowest temperature stability:

BEST FOR HOT USE	BEST FOR COLD USE
Lard, duck fat, tallow	Extra-virgin olive oil
Ghee	Macadamia oil
Macadamia oil	Avocado oil
Avocado oil	Sesame oil
Coconut oil	Hazelnut oil
Sesame oil	Almond/walnut oil
Olive oil	Flaxseed oil
Almond/walnut oil	Butter
Butter	Unrefined coconut oil

NUTS & SEEDS

Nuts and seeds are great for snacking and cooking with. However, as well as lots of healthy fats, vitamins and minerals, most nuts and seeds are high in pro-inflammatory omega-6 fatty acids and anti-nutrients such as phytic acid, which prevents mineral absorption in the body. This doesn't mean they're bad but rather that you should try to learn about the nutritional content of different nuts and seeds and consume them in moderation. You should also soak nuts and seeds for 6–12 hours and then dehydrate them back in sunlight, a dehydrator or in an oven, which removes a high per centage of anti-nutrients. The table below shows the nuts and seeds that should be consumed least and in moderation based on their nutritional, fatty acids profile and anti-nutrients content.

BEST	IN MODERATION	SMALL AMOUNTS
Macadamia nuts	Almonds	Pumpkin Seeds
Coconut, dried	Linseed	Walnuts
Chestnuts	Pistachios	Pine Nuts
Hazelnuts	Cashews	Sunflower Seeds
Flaxseeds	Brazil nuts	Sesame Seeds
Chia Seeds	Pecans	

LIQUIDS

BEST

Water

Mineral water

Coconut milk and cream

Coconut water

Almond milk, fresh if possible

Herbal teas

Kefir (fermented dairy drink)

Kombucha (fermented tea)

Bone broth, natural meat and vegetable stock

Vegetable juice

IN MODERATION

Black coffee, black tea

Low-sugar wine, sparkling wine, clear non-grain spirits such as vodka or tequila.

Small amounts of freshly squeezed juices

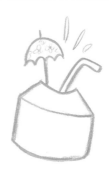

DAIRY

Consumption of dairy is a contentious topic in paleo circles. Most agree that full-fat dairy, especially from grass-fed cattle, contains many essential nutrients and fats. However, dairy also contains lactose and casein protein, and is highly insulinogenic, which makes it problematic for people with metabolic and digestive issues. A common recommendation when transitioning to a paleo diet is to avoid all dairy for thirty days. After the elimination period you can slowly re-introduce it and monitor if all or some dairy products cause any minor or major reactions in your body. If you feel better without, then it's best avoided.

I belong to the more relaxed paleo group and I include select dairy products in my dishes. I avoid plain milk but I do love butter, which is almost all fat, a little full-fat yoghurt and aged cheeses. As with most foods, not all dairy is created equal. Raw, fermented, full-fat dairy is best but it's not always easily accessible. I always look for organic, hormone- and antibiotic-free full-fat dairy from grass-fed cattle. No low-fat yoghurt, plastic cheese and skimmed milk for me!

The following dairy products are considered more superior in a paleo diet based on their nutritional profile:

BEST

Ghee	Goat & sheep's cheese, milk and yoghurt
Butter	Aged cheeses – Cheddar, Parmesan, Pecorino
Kefir	Ricotta
Full-fat, unsweetened yoghurt	Haloumi, especially from goat or sheep's milk
Cream	Feta, especially goat or sheep's milk

ADD SOME FLAVOUR

I use most fresh and dried herbs and spices, including lemongrass, kaffir lime leaves, garlic, ginger, galangal, fresh turmeric, lavender, fresh vanilla bean and horseradish. I choose good quality sea salt or Celtic salt for seasoning. I avoid pre-mixed spices and herbs that contain additives and preservatives and make my own instead.

I use these common condiments in my paleo cooking: anchovies and anchovy paste, apple sauce, capers, sun-dried tomatoes, gherkins, olives, tahini, coconut milk, coconut cream and coconut butter, fish sauce, chilli sauce, coconut aminos (similar to sweet soy sauce), most vinegars except for malt vinegar, verjuice, mustard, truffles, truffle oil, dried wild mushrooms, tomato paste, raw cacao, cocoa powder and carob powder. When buying ready-made pesto and sauces, I choose varieties with most natural ingredients and avoid anything made with soybean, canola or other vegetable oils and added sugar. Occasionally, I will use a wheat-free, gluten-fee, naturally brewed soy sauce or tamari, but not very often.

SWEET THINGS

For occasional use, I use the following natural sweeteners: raw honey, maple syrup (grade B), molasses, dark chocolate, coconut syrup/nectar, coconut sugar, green leaf stevia, apple sauce, dates, prunes, dried apricots, dried figs, palm sugar, fresh fruit juices, raw sugar and brown sugar.

WHAT ABOUT BAKING?

When it comes to baking, the following flours and meals can be used instead of standard flour: tapioca flour, chestnut flour, coconut flour, plantain flour, almond meal and flour, hazelnut meal, macadamia meal or flour, potato starch, gluten-free baking powder, baking soda, vegetable powders, ground nuts, and shredded or desiccated coconut. You can also use fresh sweet potato, pumpkin, carrots, bananas, avocados and other fruit, eggs and coconut cream in baking.

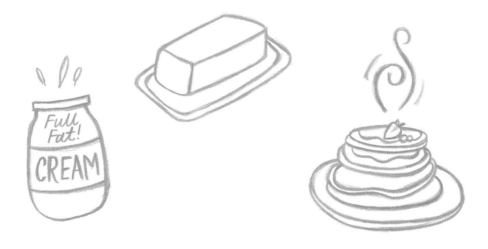

what's out

The bad news is that you will have to say goodbye to foods that until now might have been on top of your shopping list. Don't worry, you'll never go hungry without bread, beans and pasta and will be surprised at the variety of meals you can prepare without the following ingredients.

GRAINS & LEGUMES

Despite a popular belief that grains, especially whole grains, are good for us, the paleo diet advocates a complete avoidance of grains, including wheat, barley, rice and corn. Legumes are also avoided as they share similar negative properties, outlined below.

♥ *Many grains contain gluten, a complex of proteins that can cause gut inflammation and damage to the gut lining, leading to malabsoprtion of nutrients. Gluten has also been associated with such conditions and symptoms as gastrointestinal issues, skin problems, autoimmune disease and mental health issues.*

♥ *Grains and legumes are high in carbohydrates. The paleo diet is not against carbohydrates per se but it does advocate a low-to-moderate intake, which is more suitable to modern lifestyles. Consuming more carbohydrates than your body needs can lead to problems such as insulin resistance, obesity, type 2 diabetes and some cancers.*

♥ *They also contain anti-nutrients – natural or synthetic compounds that inhibit the absorption of nutrients – such as phytic acid and lectins. Phytic acid, or phytates, is found in plant-based foods, most prevalently in grains and legumes, and in moderate amounts in nuts and seeds. It prevents the absorption of some minerals into the bloodstream, and mineral deficiency has been linked to issues such as osteoporosis, skin conditions, muscle cramping, fatigue, poor immunity and more. It's best to limit its consumption by avoiding grains and legumes and soaking nuts and seeds before usage.*

♥ *Lectins are found in most plant-based foods and are especially high in grains and legumes. Lectins are a naturally occurring defence mechanism of some plants that protect their survival by irritating the digestive system of mammals consuming it, including us. Such damage to the gut lining impairs the absorption of nutrients.*

To play devil's advocate, I would like to point out that some ancient cultures consumed wild grains such as wild rice and corn. The difference between now and then is in the amounts, level of processing and the methods of cooking and preparation. The Weston A. Price Foundation dietary philosophy, based on studies of ancient cultures and their health, recommends fermentation, soaking and cooking methods to improve the nutritional profile of certain grains and legumes and to remove some of the anti-nutrients.

Grains and legumes to avoid include, but are not limited to, the following:

GRAINS	LEGUMES	PSEUDOGRAINS
Wheat	Soy beans	Quinoa
Barley	Black eyed beans	Amaranth
Rye	Red kidney beans	Chia seeds
Corn (maize)	Cannellini beans	Buckwheat
Spelt	Dried peas	Hemp
Bran	Split peas	Flax
Polenta	Lentils	
Millet	Chickpeas	
Oats	Buttter beans	
Kamut	Borlotti beans	
Brown/wild/white rice	Pinto beans	
Sorghum		

♥ *According to the Perfect Health Diet, white rice is essentially a carbohydrate with neither nutrients nor toxins, so although it's high in carbohydrates, it won't do much harm if consumed in small amounts.*

♥ *Legumes have to be soaked, fermented or sprouted to make them safe to eat. For convenience, most choose to simply avoid them. Soy beans and soy products, such as soy milk, tofu and meat substitutes, are most harmful and should be avoided, while some fermented soy foods, such as miso, nato and naturally brewed wheat- and gluten-free soy sauce, can be eaten occasionally.*

♥ *Pseudograins contain similar anti-nutrient properties to grains and legumes; however, as they're typically comprised of more proteins, B vitamins, iron and healthy fatty acids, they're considered more nutritious and safer to eat. Pseudograins can be consumed occasionally if handled properly – soaked and washed before cooking.*

PROCESSED, REFINED, ARTIFICIAL SUGAR & SWEETENERS

I'm sure this is not the first time you'll read that too much sugar is not good for you. The list of sugar 'achievements' is long and well documented – it's linked to overeating, hypoglycaemia, obesity, diabetes, digestive problems, and the development of multiple cancers. But sweeteners aren't all bad. The nutritional value of sweeteners depends on how they're made, where they're used and how our body processes them. Here is a breakdown of sugars and sweeteners that should be avoided (that includes drinks and foods containing them).

White table sugar, icing sugar, high-fructose corn syrup, corn syrup, brown-rice malt syrup, malt syrup, beet sugar, barley malt, golden syrup, caramel, carob syrup, Demerara sugar, dextrose, fructose, grape sugar, maltose, maltodextrin, sorghum syrup, yellow sugar, xylitol, light brown sugar, agave and agave nectar (90 per cent fructose and only 10 per cent glucose). Plus such artificial sugars as aspartame (sold as NutraSweet or Equal), saccharin (Sweet n Low), sucralose (Splenda), acesulfame-K (Sunette or Sweet One) and sorbitol.

VEGETABLE & SEED OILS

While naturally occurring, minimally processed fats and oils (such as olive oil and butter) are a healthy source of energy and nutrients, highly processed vegetable and seed oils (such as soybean, canola and corn oil) contain high levels of omega-6 fatty acids, which – when consumed in excess – have detrimental health effects. Problem is – these oils are present in nearly everything we eat nowadays. Grain-fed livestock, where a lot of meat produce comes from, is also high in omega-6. A diet high in omega-6 is associated with an increase in inflammatory diseases such as cardiovascular disease, type 2 diabetes, rheumatoid arthritis, asthma and cancer to mention a few.

In addition to omega-6 fatty acids, most polyunsaturated oils are highly prone to oxidation and rancidity, which turns these so-called 'heart healthy' oils to toxic liquids. For these reasons, it's best to avoid the following fats and oils: corn, cottonseed, soybean, canola, safflower, sunflower, peanut, grape seed, vegetable and margarine, which is made from aforementioned oils.

A NOTE ON PROCESSED FOODS

Transitioning into paleo, I became very aware of how many processed foods – aka anything that comes in a package, bottle or a can – and by default, many restaurant meals, contain toxic ingredients such as gluten, processed sugars and industrial oils. Much of the time you simply have to turn a blind eye to what oils and additives are used in meal preparation or you would have no social life. Depending on where you live, you can find products and brands that use mostly natural ingredients and ethical practices. For everything else, it's all about reading the labels. Cooking for yourself and your family is the ability to control what goes into your food.

And that's pretty much it, my friends. Before we get cooking, let me show you what I have in my kitchen and fridge to create an easy-peasy paleo cooking experience.

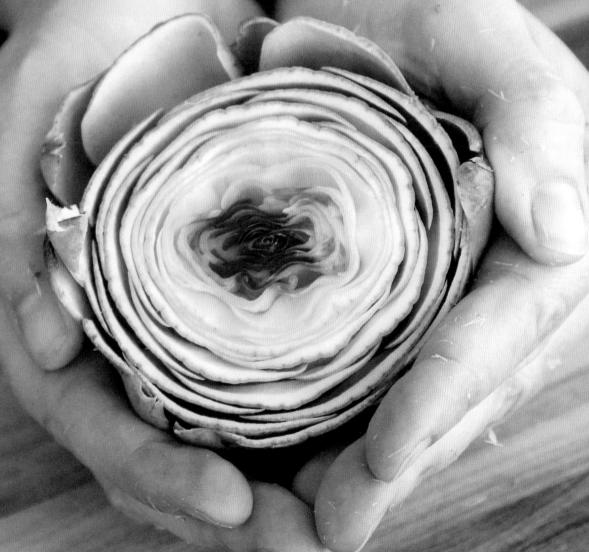

KITCHEN
BASICS

Little things
A few chopping boards, spatula, can opener, colander, fine-mesh sieve, grater, hand held whisk, kettle, ladle, lemon juicer, Mason jars, meat mallet, measuring jug, mortar and pestle, pastry brush, peeler, potato masher, rolling pin, tongs, salad spinner, scales, slotted spoon, wooden spoon.

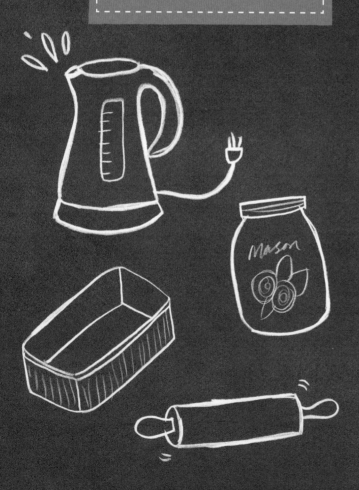

Dutch oven/casserole *Cook curries, roasts, braised meats, tagines and soups. I use a large, heavy-lidded Le Creuset.*

Food processor *Chop, slice, grate, grind, blend and purée in seconds.*

Electric standing blender
Purée and blend soups, smoothies and condiments.

Hand electric mixer
Whip, whisk and blend; choose a five-speed model.

Slow cooker *The ultimate magic pot! Cook large batches of braised meats, casseroles, tagines and soups with minimum effort.*

Round cake tin/spring-form tin
Bake frittatas, sponge cakes, pies and layered dishes.

Loaf tin *Make banana bread, meat loaf and terrines.*

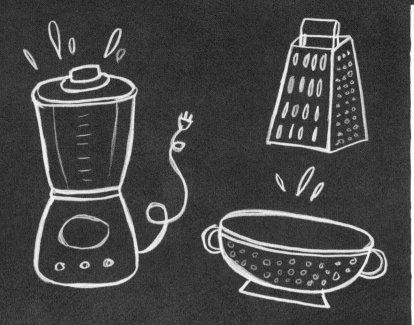

Thermometer (dial or digital) *Check the doneness of roast meats and measure liquid temperature.*

Barbecue or a chargrill pan *Chargrill meats, seafood or vegetables.*

Wok *Make quick stir-fries and fried cauliflower rice.*

Mandolin *Slice fruit and vegetables into really thin slices and ribbons.*

Juicer *I love vegetable juices, to drink and to cook with.*

Storage containers *Mixed-size glass or steel containers to store your kitchen prep and leftovers.*

Muffin tin *I use for egg muffins, cupcakes and mini meat pies.*

Flat oven tray x 2 *Bake cookies, dehydrate nuts, beef jerky and oven-dried tomatoes.*

Large roasting tray x 2 *Use for roast meats, vegetables, lasagne and large casserole bakes.*

Small saucepan *Boil eggs, make sauces, melted chocolate, soups.*

Medium saucepan *Make sauces, cook vegetables and soups.*

Large saucepan *Cook large vegetables, master stocks and sterilise jars.*

Small frying pan *Pan-fry eggs and bacon, omelettes, sauté vegetables, thicken sauces.*

Large frying pan with deep sides *Pan-fry meat, sear roasts, cook stews, vegetables and meatballs.*

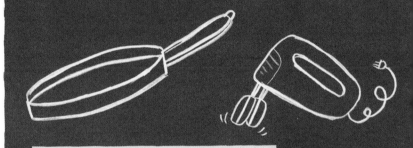

OPTIONAL: Fancy-schmancy tools everyone raves about

Thermomix *Superhero appliance that can chop, beat, mix, cook, melt, emulsify, weigh, knead and stir.*

Magic Bullet *A mini blender you can throw in your suitcase.*

Dehydrator *Dry out soaked nuts, make dried fruit and beef jerky.*

Bento-style lunch containers and a thermos

in my pantry

I usually keep the following foods and ingredients in my pantry.
Many of these will move in to the fridge after opening.

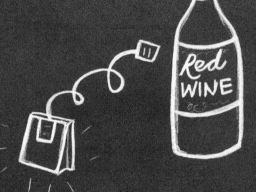

Dry goodies
A collection of teas and coffee beans, almond meal, almonds, cashews, coconut flour, coconut syrup or coconut sugar, dark chocolate, gluten-free baking powder, macadamia nuts, natural stevia, pumpkin seeds, quinoa and white rice (for THOSE days), raw cacao powder, sesame seeds, tapioca flour, vanilla extract.

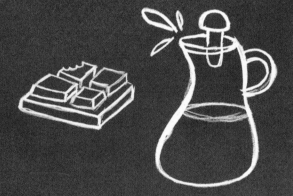

Liquids & condiments
Apple cider vinegar, balsamic vinegar, coconut aminos, coconut butter , coconut milk, coconut oil, coconut water, fish sauce, gluten-free Worcestershire sauce, hot chilli sauce, macadamia oil, mustard, raw honey, red wine, sesame oil, tahini, verjuice, virgin olive oil, extra-virgin olive oil, white wine vinegar.

Spices & dried herbs
Bay leaves, black pepper, chilli flakes, cinnamon, cloves, coriander seed powder, cumin powder, curry powder, five-spice powder, garlic powder, Italian herbs, nutmeg, rosemary leaves, sea salt or Celtic salt, smoked paprika, star anise, sweet paprika, turmeric.

Jars & tins
Anchovies, artichokes, capers, gherkins, horseradish, jalapenos, salmon, sardines, sun-dried tomatoes, tinned tomatoes, tomato paste.

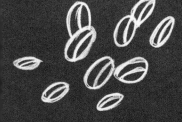

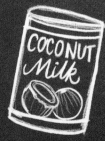

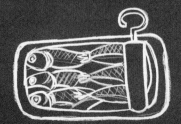

in my fridge

An inventory of fresh food in our house depends on the season and events but on a typical day, after a big weekly or fortnightly shop, you will find the following in my kitchen fridge and on my countertop.

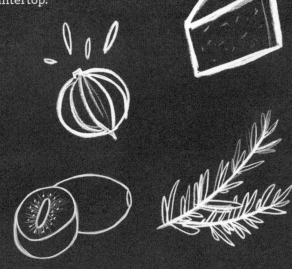

Fresh produce
A mix of fresh herbs, apples, avocados, bananas, berries, broccoli, cabbage, carrots, cauliflower, celery, cucumber, tomatoes, cucumber, garlic, ginger, kiwifruit, mixed lettuce, mushrooms, onion, pumpkin, radishes, red peppers, spinach, sweet potato, tomatoes.

Freezer
Frozen berries, frozen soup, frozen spinach, frozen stock cubes, green peas, sausages.

Fats
Butter, ghee, fish oil.

Protein
Free-range bacon, cooked prawns, free-range eggs, Greek, full-fat yoghurt or coconut yoghurt, lamb chops or shanks, liver pâté, minced beef, olives, Parmesan and haloumi cheese, salami, sauerkraut, whole chicken.

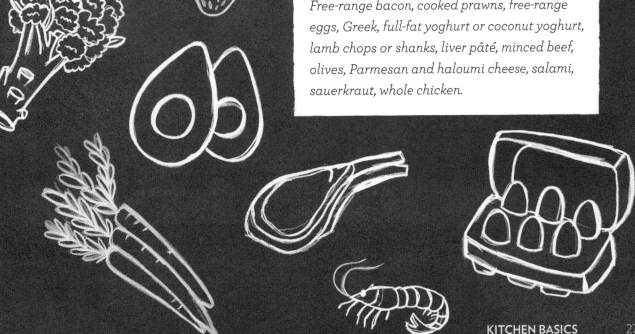

— my favourite —
blogs & websites

♥ **AUSTRALIA**

Eat Sleep Move

Indi Nature

Lady Homemade

Modern Paleo

Nourishing Australia

Paleo Foodies

Paleo in Melbourne

Rejuvenated For Life

Sarah Wilson

Pete Evans

The Healthy Chef

The Merrymaker Sisters

The Paleo Network

What Katie Ate

♥ **AROUND THE WORLD**

Lookbook Cookbook

PaleoDish (Canada)

Paleo Britain

Paleo Polly

Swiss Paleo

Strictly Paleo-ish (Sweden)

The Fitness Explorer

♥ **USA**

Against All Grain

Balanced Bites

Cave Girl Eats

Chris Kresser

Civilized Caveman

Clothes Make The Girl

Elana's Pantry

Everyday Paleo

Living Paleo

Mark's Daily Apple

Nom Nom Paleo

Paleo Cupboard

Paleo OMG

Paleo Parents

Primal Palate

Primal Toad

Robb Wolf

Rubies & Radishes

The Domestic Man

The Kitchn

The Paleo Mum

Wellness Mama

Weston A Price

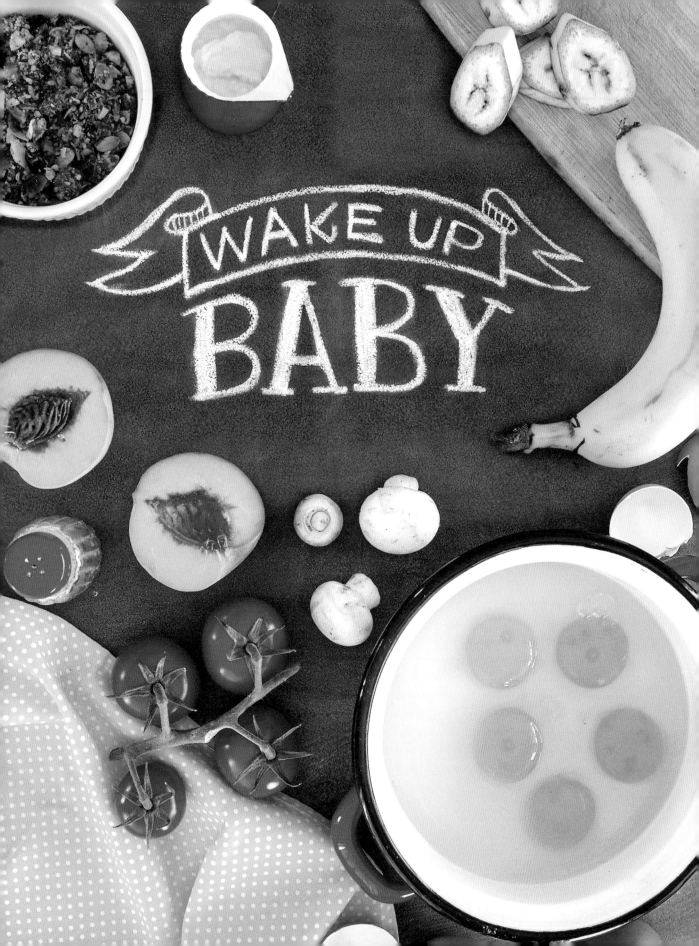

hazelnut pancakes with blood orange sauce

What better way to start a Sunday than with a sleep-in and batch of fluffy pancakes with freshly brewed coffee. These paleo pancakes have a slightly different texture but people I've made them for prefer them to standard pancakes.

MAKES 12 PANCAKES

For the sauce

60g butter

3 blood oranges (1 juiced, 2 peeled and sliced)

Juice from 1 orange

1 tbsp lemon juice

2 tsp coconut sugar or raw honey

1 vanilla bean, sliced in half

For the pancakes

4 eggs

1 tsp vanilla extract/essence

1 banana

2 tbsp coconut flour

165g hazelnut meal

1/2 tsp baking soda/bicarb soda (or gluten–free baking powder)

Ghee or coconut oil for cooking

For the sauce, heat butter in a small saucepan. Add blood orange juice and orange juice, lemon juice, coconut sugar and fresh vanilla bean. Bring to simmer and add slices of blood orange. Cook on low heat for 15 minutes, stirring occasionally.

Meanwhile, whisk eggs and vanilla extract in a bowl. Mash banana and fold into the liquid mixture. Add flour and hazelnut meal and sprinkle baking soda all over the mix. Whisk until well combined.

A simpler method is to blend all ingredients in a blender. Add liquid ingredients and banana first and, after ten seconds of blending, add the dry ingredients and whizz a few times.

Heat a large frying pan over medium heat and melt a teaspoon of ghee or coconut oil. Using about a quarter of a cup of mixture per pancake, cook the first batch for 2 minutes on one side, or until bubbles appear on the surface, and for another minute on the other side. Transfer to a plate and cover loosely with aluminum foil or a towel to keep warm. Repeat with the remaining mixture, brushing pan with extra ghee in between batches. Serve drizzled with blood orange sauce.

If you don't have enough time to make the sauce, serve pancakes with berries, banana and some raw honey. If avoiding butter, use two tablespoons of ghee or coconut oil instead. Almond meal can be used instead of hazelnut meal.

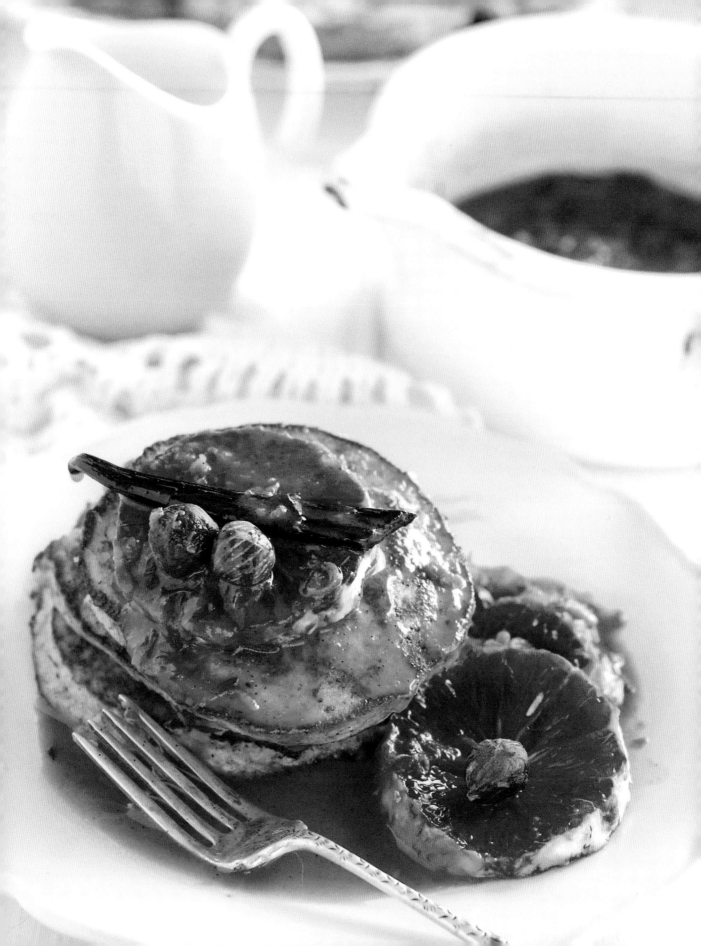

breakfast granola

We make this granola almost every week, as it's a perfect alternative to eggs and can be taken in a zip-lock bag as a snack on the go. I usually have 50 grams of granola with some natural yoghurt and berries but you can also have it with coconut or almond milk and other non-dairy yoghurts.

MAKES 10 SERVINGS

500g mixed almonds, hazelnuts and macadamia nuts

100g dried plums or dried cherries, cranberries or apricots

70g pumpkin seeds

70g desiccated coconut

45g coconut flakes (or add more desiccated coconut)

2 tbsp maple syrup

2–3 tbsp honey or coconut syrup

1 tsp vanilla extract

Zest of 1 orange (optional)

Coconut oil

1–2 tbsp chia seeds

Ideally, you should start this recipe by 'activating' the nuts and seeds you plan to use in the granola. Learn how to do it on the Eat Drink Paleo website. Alternatively, use raw nuts as they are, but they will contain some phytic acid.

Preheat oven to 170°C (335°F). In a food processor, grind 400g of nuts and dried fruit to smaller crumbs. Some of it will turn into finer flour/meal-like consistency but that's what we want – a variety of shapes and sizes. Mix processed nuts with the remaining whole nuts and the other ingredients, except for the chia seeds and coconut oil in a large mixing bowl. Use a wooden spoon or a spatula to break down the clumps forming from maple syrup and honey coming into contact with dry ingredients. Some of it can remain unbroken.

Grease a deep oven tray with coconut oil and line with baking paper, making sure the sides are covered. Spoon the mixture into the tray and flatten with a spatula. Bake for 10 minutes, then mix through to expose the bottom layer of granola to the heat before baking for a further 8–10 minutes. Stir again and bake for the final 3–4 minutes.

Once browned, remove and let it cool completely. Add chia seeds and transfer to an airtight container. It will last for about two weeks in a pantry and longer if kept refrigerated.

Enjoy with coconut yoghurt from page 182.

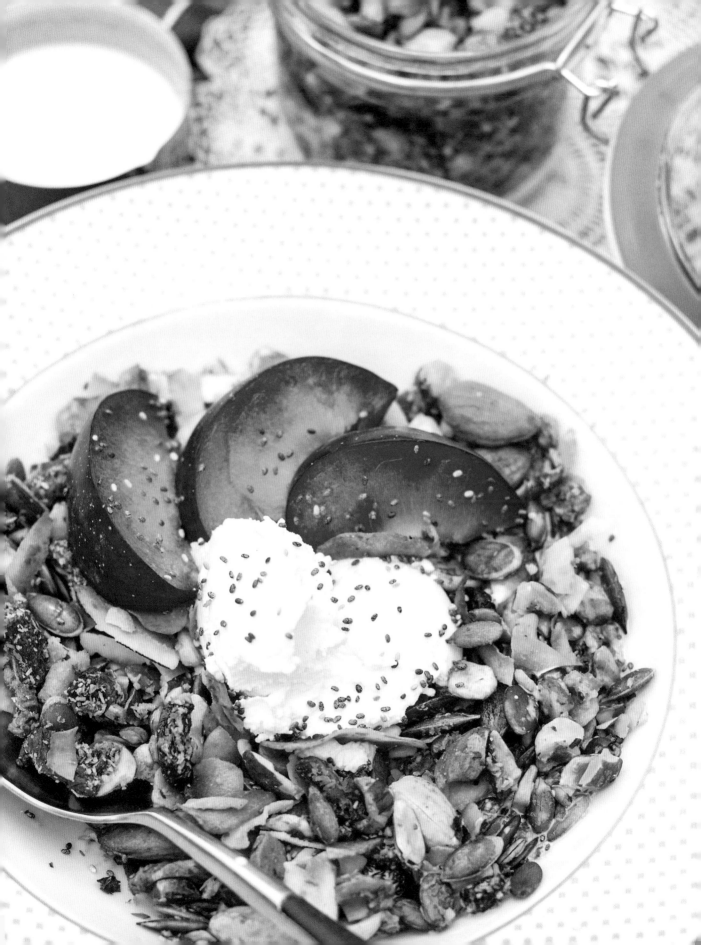

asparagus soldiers eggs & truffle

Ever since I was a little girl I loved eggs and soldiers. These days, as I don't eat bread, I use whatever else I can find to dip into a creamy, nutritious egg yolk. Using asparagus sautéed in some butter and truffle oil takes the whole experience to the next level.

SERVES 2

4 medium eggs

12 asparagus spears, ends trimmed

1 tsp virgin olive oil or butter

1 tsp truffle oil

Squeeze of lemon juice or a little dash of verjuice

Sea salt and pepper

Truffle-infused oil is usually made with extra-virgin oil that's been infused with truffle mushrooms. Invest in a small bottle from your local deli and it will last you for ages. Add to scrambled eggs, mashed cauliflower, roasted mushrooms, steak sauces and salad dressings. Verjuice is a highly acidic juice made by pressing unripe grapes. It can be used in place of vinegar or lemon juice.

Take eggs out of the fridge, if that's where you keep them, 5–10 minutes before cooking to bring them to room temperature. Bring a small saucepan with enough water to cover the eggs to boil. Take off the heat once boiling. Place eggs in a slotted spoon and gently lower to the bottom of the saucepan. Leave eggs to settle for 10 seconds and then place the saucepan back on the heat to bring back to boil. Set the timer for 5 minutes for a soft centre and firm whites. Place cooked eggs under cold running water for 15 seconds to stop cooking and to make peeling easier.

Sometimes the eggs can crack in boiling water. Some recommend pricking the bigger end of the egg with a needle before immersing it in the water. I find that placing them in a saucepan while off the heat prevents them from rolling around in boiling bubbles and bringing the eggs to room temperature before cooking means they're not too cold when going into boiling water. The cooking time will differ if you have larger or smaller eggs or if you live at higher altitude. The higher you are above sea level the longer you have to cook the egg for the same effect.

While eggs are cooking, pan-fry asparagus spears in butter and truffle oil on medium heat for 1–2 minutes and sprinkle with a little sea salt and pepper.

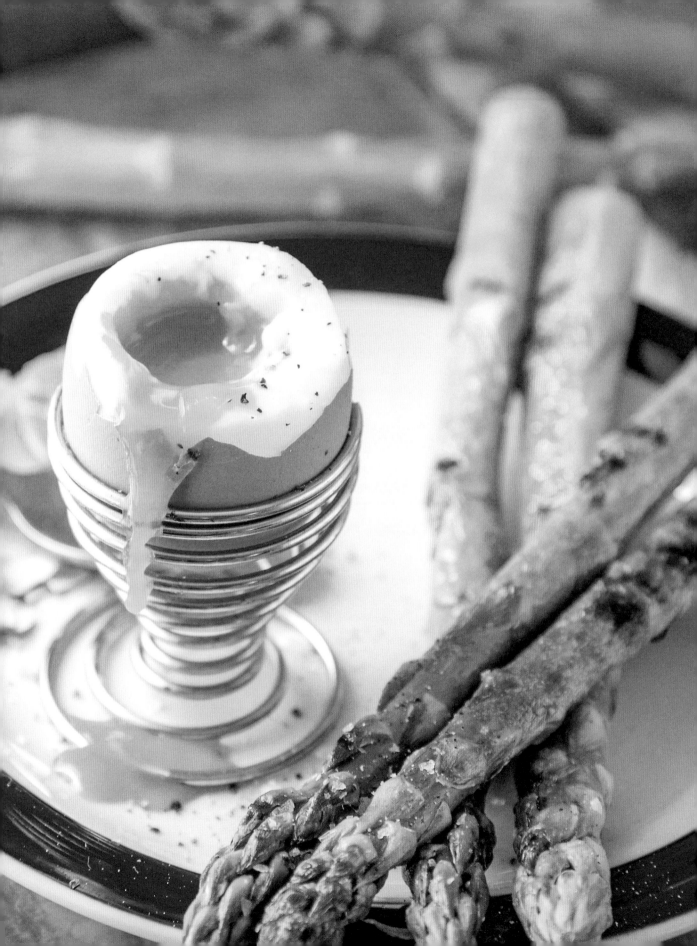

velvet summer quiche

Velvet summer is that period when summer crosses into autumn, when the nights get cold but the day sun is still warm and feels like velvet on your skin. It's the time you get back into comfort food and baking. The flavours and texture of this quiche remind me of that gorgeous time of year.

SERVES 4–6

Macadamia/coconut oil or ghee for cooking

1 large sweet potato, diced

2 brown onions, sliced

1 red pepper, sliced

2 tbsp fresh thyme leaves

5 garlic cloves, finely chopped

1 tbsp balsamic vinegar

Pinch of sea salt

10 eggs

180ml double cream (can be omitted)

Zest of 1 lemon

Sea salt and pepper for seasoning

45g grated Parmesan or cheddar cheese

50g pine nuts

Preheat oven to 200°C (390°F). Grease a flat baking tray with coconut oil and scatter diced sweet potato. Bake for 20 minutes. Remove and turn the oven down to 180°C (355°F), ready for the quiche to go in.

In a medium frying pan, sauté onion and red peppers in ghee or macadamia oil on medium heat for 15 minutes. After 10 minutes of cooking, add fresh thyme, garlic, balsamic vinegar and a pinch of salt.

Whisk eggs with cream and combine with the lemon zest, a pinch of black pepper, a generous pinch of sea salt and grated cheese. Grease the bottom of a deep baking tray with coconut oil and line with baking paper, making sure the sides are covered. Assemble sweet potatoes and onion and red peppers mix evenly on the bottom. Pour whisked egg mix on top. Bake for 10 minutes, then sprinkle with pine nuts and some extra fresh thyme and bake for a further 15 minutes. Stand aside to cool and settle for 5 minutes before serving. Lift the sides of baking paper to remove the quiche to a cutting board before slicing and serving.

You can use a round baking tin instead. If avoiding dairy, make without cream and cheese, although the quiche will lack the creaminess and fluffy texture of a standard quiche. The quiche will keep for up to 3–4 days in the fridge. Cream and cheddar cheese can be omitted, replace with an extra egg or two.

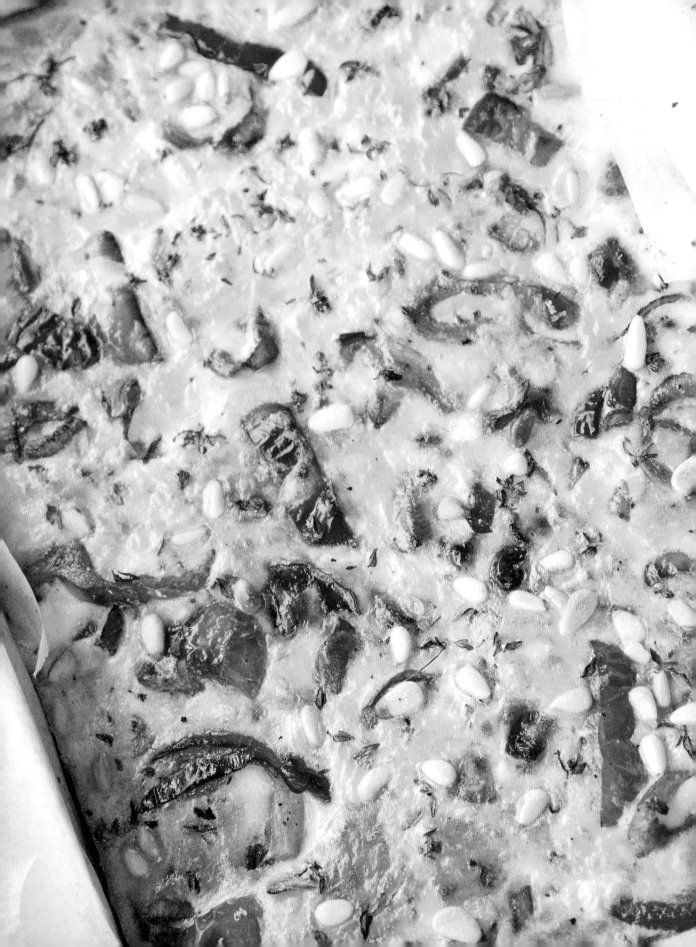

banana bread

This banana bread is super easy to make and tastes just as good as the regular wheat flour version. I make it a lot as it's very handy to have a few slices around for snacks, packed lunches, travel and on-the-go breakfasts.

SERVES 10

Coconut oil

3 eggs

Pinch of salt

2 bananas, mashed

1 tbsp raw honey or maple syrup

1 tsp vanilla extract

2 1/2 tbsp coconut oil or macadamia oil

165g cups almond meal

1 tsp gluten-free baking powder

3 tbsp of tapioca flour

Pinch of nutmeg

1 tsp of cinnamon

2 tbsp desiccated coconut

2–3 tbsp walnuts, chopped

50g diced dried apricots or figs

Preheat oven to 165°C (330°F). Brush a loaf tin with coconut oil and line the bottom with non-stick baking paper.

Method 1: Place eggs with a pinch of salt in a large mixing bowl and whisk until thick and foamy. Add mashed banana, honey, vanilla and coconut oil, and whisk together until well incorporated.

Add almond meal, baking powder, tapioca, nutmeg, cinnamon and desiccated coconut, and mix together well. Fold in walnuts and dried fruit and pour the batter into the prepared tin. Smooth the surface and place a few walnuts on the top.

Method 2: Place eggs, banana, honey, vanilla, coconut oil and a pinch of salt in a blender and whiz for 20–30 seconds until thick and foamy. Then add the remaining ingredients except for the walnuts and apricots and blend until smooth and thick, scraping the sides along the way. Fold in walnuts and dried apricots and continue as in method one.

Bake for 45–55 minutes on the middle shelf. Insert a bamboo skewer into the centre to see if it comes out dry, in which case it's done. Remove from the oven and let it cool for 5–10 minutes before removing from the tin. Cover with a towel if leaving overnight. Serve as is or toast and smother with some butter.

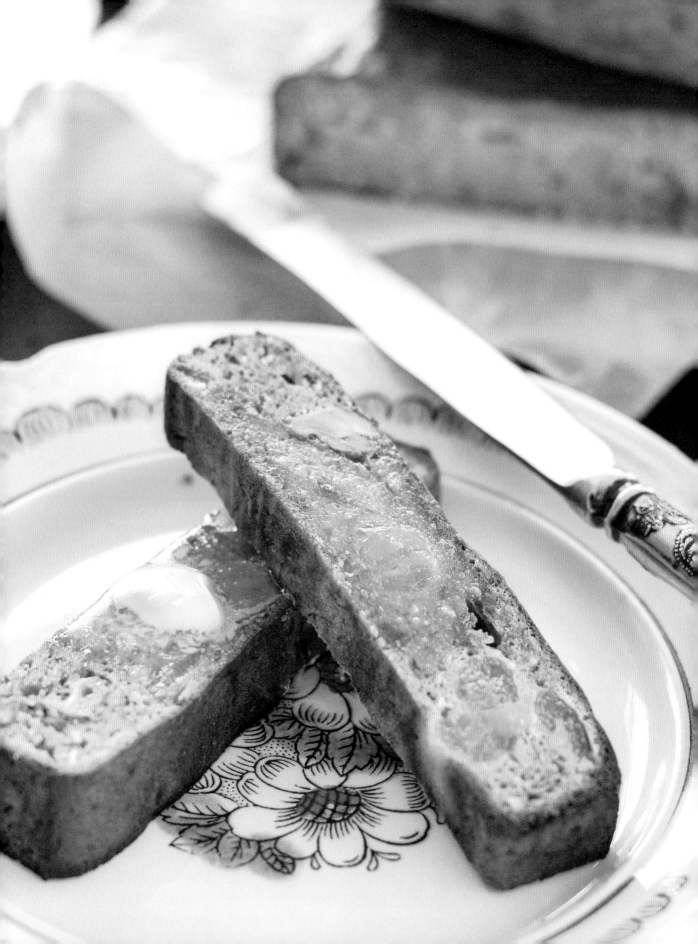

harissa chorizo egg crepes

This recipe was a bit of an accident. I was tossing up between savoury crepes and a Mexican breakfast burrito. This is what I ended up with and luckily it was so delicious, it made it to the cookbook.

SERVES 2

2 tbsp olive oil

1/2 Spanish onion, finely diced

1/2 red pepper, finely diced

1 medium chorizo sausage

1 tbsp harissa (see page 176)

6 eggs

Pinch of salt

Ghee for cooking egg crepes

Fresh coriander and avocado to serve

Heat olive oil in a small frying pan. Sauté onion and red peppers for 3–4 minutes or until softened.

Meanwhile, peel the skin off chorizo and cut in chunks. Grind to a mince in a food processor or finely dice with a knife. Add to onion and red pepper, together with harissa, and cook for 3–4 minutes until browned and slightly caramelised. Remove to a bowl.

Whisk eggs with a pinch of salt. Preheat a frying pan with half a teaspoon of ghee on medium heat for 30 seconds. Ladle just enough egg mixture to coat the bottom of the pan. Using the handle, swirl the egg around to form a thin crepe–like pancake. Cook for 1 minute. Run a spatula around the outside of the crepe as it cooks to loosen it. Gently lift the crepe up and flip it over (you might not even need to do that if it's thin enough to cook through from the bottom). Slide the crepe onto a plate and repeat with the remaining mixture.

Fold a couple of tablespoons of cooked chorizo mixture inside the crepe like in a parcel and serve with fresh coriander and slices of avocado.

Chorizo is a smoked Spanish sausage made with pork and lots of paprika, garlic and other spices. Look for good quality chorizo made with natural ingredients. Harissa is a spicy chilli sauce originating in northern Africa. Make it yourself or use a good quality store-bought harissa.

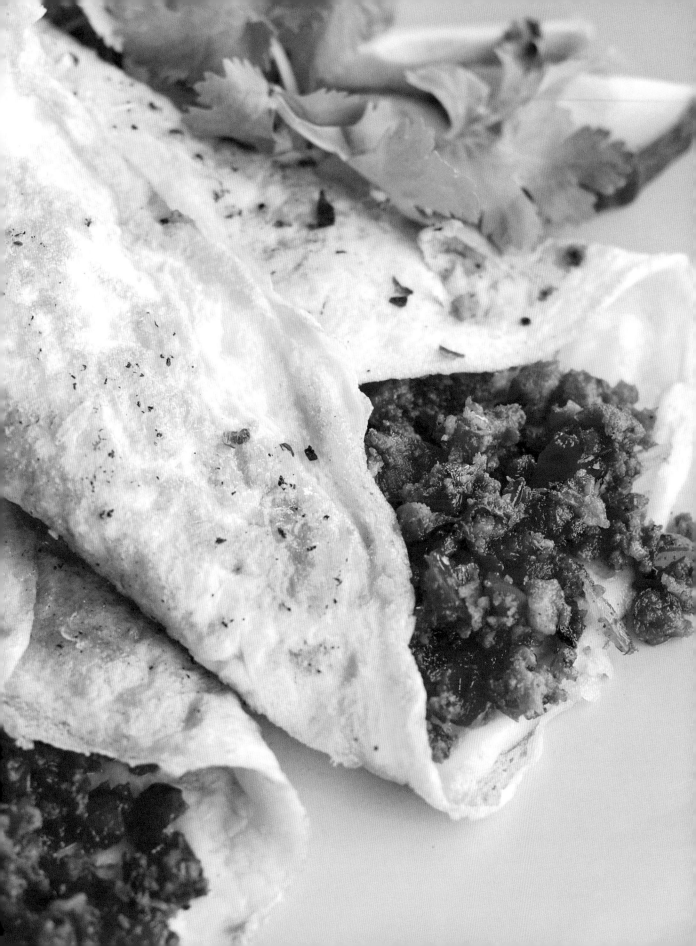

chai banana porridge

Warm and nourishing, this porridge is a real treat that tastes like something you might have at a yoga retreat in India. Save it for the weekend when you have time to enjoy it slowly.

SERVES 2

65g blanched macadamia nuts

75g blanched almonds

1 banana

250ml coconut milk

125ml water

45g desiccated coconut

1 tbsp chia seeds

1/2 tsp ground cardamom

1/2 tsp ground ginger

1/2 tsp cinnamon

Pinch of ground nutmeg

Pinch of salt

1 tsp vanilla extract

1 tbsp raw honey to drizzle over

Fresh berries and cinnamon
to serve

In a food processor, grind macadamia nuts and almonds into small crumbs. Add banana and process together until banana is puréed. Alternatively, you can use a fork to mash the banana and a mortar and pestle to break the nuts. Transfer to a small saucepan.

Add the rest of ingredients, except honey. Bring to simmer and cook for a couple of minutes. Serve in bowls drizzled with honey, fresh berries and some cinnamon.

To speed up the process, you can keep a larger batch of processed nuts mixed with spices in a jar in the pantry, ready to go. Blanched nuts refers to nuts with no skin on. You can easily use regular almonds.

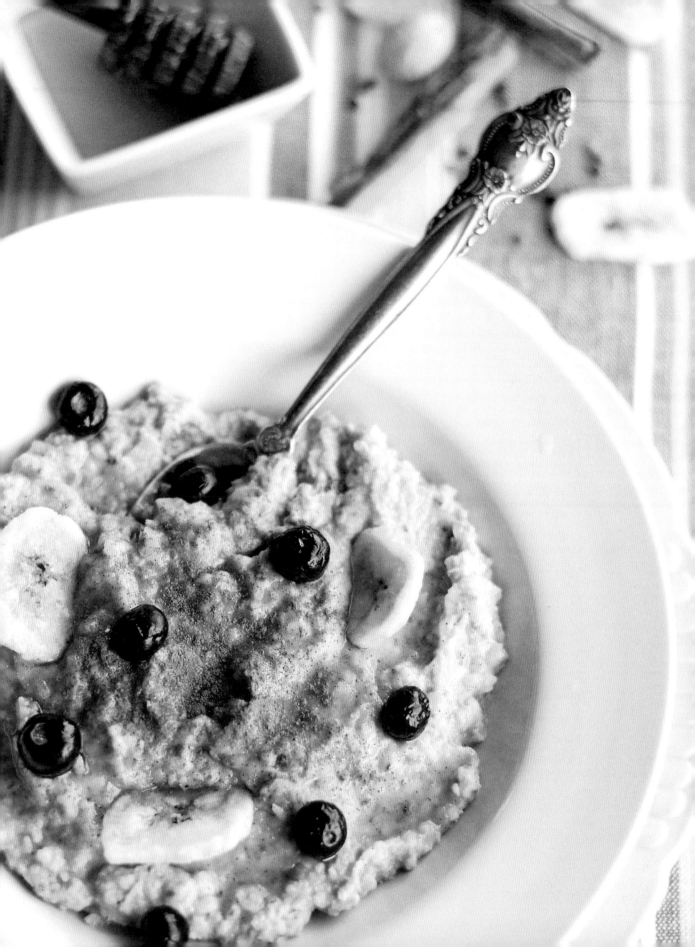

courgette & bacon fritters

Fancy a little café breakfast at home? You can't go past tasty, filling fritters.
Make a bigger batch and have some for the next day's lunch and snacks.
Kids will love them too.

SERVES 3

For the onion relish

3 tbsp virgin olive oil

2 medium brown onions, sliced

1 long red chilli, finely diced

2/3 tsp sea salt

1 garlic clove, finely chopped

2 tbsp balsamic vinegar

1 tbsp tomato paste

1/2 tsp coriander seed powder

125ml water

For the fritters

2 rashers of bacon, diced and trimmed of excess fat

Ghee for cooking

2 medium green courgettes, grated (discard the middle with seeds)

1 medium carrot, peeled and grated

1/2 chopped spring onion

2 eggs

2 tbsp tapioca flour

2/3 tsp sea salt

1/2 tsp pepper

1/4 tsp gluten–free baking powder

3 tbsp coconut oil

For the relish, heat olive oil in a medium frying pan or a saucepan to hot but not sizzling. Add onion, chilli and salt and turn the heat down to low–medium. Sauté onion for 4–5 minutes, then add the rest of ingredients. Mix through and cook for 15 minutes until softened and caramelised.

Pan-fry bacon pieces in a little ghee or excess fat from the bacon until crispy. Remove to a plate with paper towel to drain some of the fat off.

In a large bowl, mix the rest of the fritter ingredients with crispy bacon into a thick, moist batter. Heat coconut oil in a large frying pan. Using a cup or a large serving spoon, scoop the batter mixture gently into the hot coconut oil, as individual patties, about 1–2cm apart. Fry for 3 minutes on each side or until a golden brown crust forms, adding more coconut oil if needed. Serve with the onion relish and some extra spring onions.

Tapioca flour can be replaced with fine almond meal, chestnut flour or potato starch. Coconut flour can also be used but it will absorb more liquid, which might result in slightly drier fritters. If avoiding nightshades, remove chilli from the relish recipe and replace with some black or white pepper for heat. You can use the leftover onion relish with grilled lamb or beefsteaks, or to fold into a frittata mixture. Leftover courgette and carrot peel can be used for a master vegetable stock.

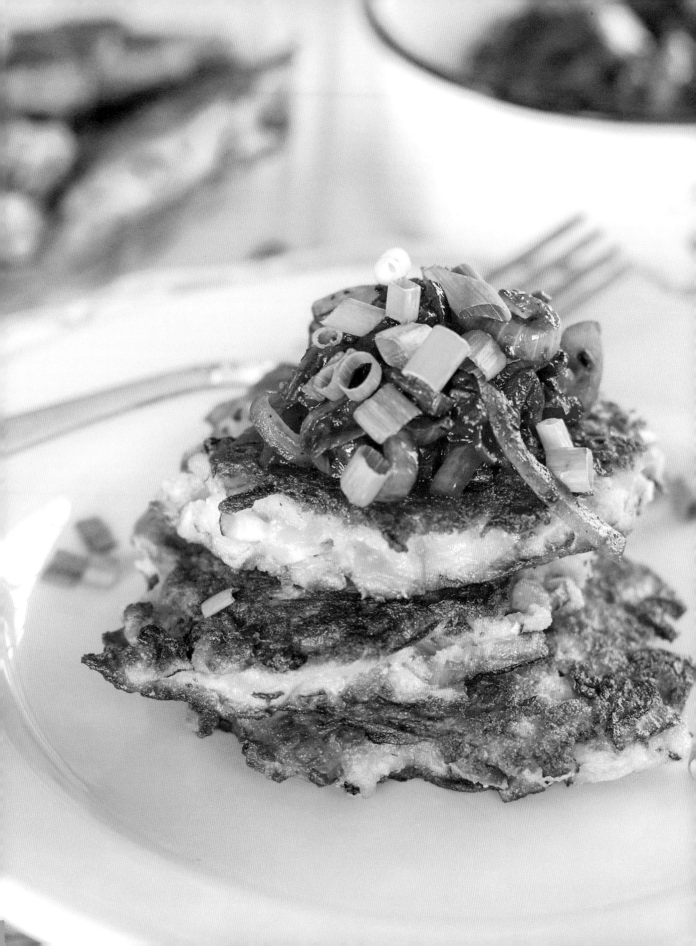

sweet potato rosti with sardines salad

Paleo breakfasts are not just about eggs. Whenever I feel as though omelette and I need a little break from each other, I turn to this other savoury favourite of mine. This dish packs a lot of energy, vitamin C, beta-carotene and omega-3 fatty acids.

SERVES 2

2 tbsp coconut oil or ghee

1 medium sweet potato, peeled and grated

2/3 tsp of sea salt

1/2 tsp of pepper

1/2 medium cucumber, sliced

1/2 fresh fennel, sliced

1/2 green apple, thinly sliced

1/2 red onion, sliced

1 tbsp chopped fresh dill

1 tbsp extra-virgin olive oil

1 tbsp lemon juice

100–150g tinned sardines

1 tbsp mayonnaise

Heat coconut oil or ghee in a medium frying pan to sizzling hot. Add grated sweet potato and flatten with a spatula. Turn the heat down to medium and cook, scraping and turning it every couple of minutes, for a total of 10 minutes. Sprinkle with sea salt and pepper.

Mix cucumber, fennel, apple, onion and dill with olive oil and lemon juice. Split open sardines and remove backbone. Assemble the mix on top of sardine fillets and serve with a side of sweet potato rosti and a dollop of mayonnaise.

Use mayonnaise made with olive oil or macadamia oil rather than standard soybean or vegetable oil based varieties. You can find a recipe for a homemade mayo on page 191. Tinned salmon or tuna can be used instead of sardines.

macadamia & artichoke stuffed mushrooms

Another egg-free recipe to add to your breakfast repertoire. You can prepare all ingredients and stuff the mushrooms the night before, so all you have to do in the morning is stick them in the oven while you're getting ready.

Soak macadamia nuts in a cup of water for 3–4 hours.

On medium heat, sauté onion in a tablespoon of ghee or olive oil until soft and golden.

Rinse the nuts and place in a food processor together with artichokes, cooked onion, garlic, lemon zest, salt, pepper and a tablespoon of ghee or butter. Process into smooth, thick paste.

Preheat oven to 180°C (355°F) and grease a flat baking tray with olive oil or ghee. Fill mushrooms with a teaspoon of artichoke paste each. Place on a greased tray and bake in the oven for 20–30 minutes. Serve with fresh parsley and crispy bacon on the side.

You could use 4–6 larger portobello mushrooms instead of smaller button mushrooms. Cashew nuts can be used instead of macadamia nuts. If you eat butter, add that to the filling instead of ghee or olive oil for richer taste.

SERVES 2

65g macadamia nuts

1 medium brown onion, diced

2 tbsp ghee or virgin olive oil

3 artichokes (from a jar)

1 garlic clove, peeled

Zest from 1 lemon

2/3 tsp sea salt

Pinch of pepper

1 tbsp ghee or virgin olive oil for cooking

12 large button mushrooms, wiped clean, stems separated from cups

Parsley and a few rashers of crispy bacon to serve

smoked salmon 'not bagel'

I've always been a big fan of bagels with smoked salmon but, since I don't eat bagels any more, I've decided to create a bagel-like sandwich using sweet potato patties. This recipe is very simple and the final result is a worthy substitute that satisfies my smoked salmon bagel cravings.

SERVES 1

1 medium sweet potato (300g)

A few pinches of sea salt

Pinch of ground black pepper

1 tbsp coconut flour

1 tbsp ghee or coconut oil for frying

1 tbsp mayonnaise

2–3 slices of smoked salmon

1/4 red onion, sliced

1 tbsp baby capers

Peel and finely grate the sweet potato. Combine with salt, pepper and coconut flour until a sticky dough forms. Heat ghee or coconut oil in a frying pan. Using your hands, mould potato mixture into two fat, round patties and place in sizzling hot fat. Flatten with a spatula and cook for 4–5 minutes on each side, on medium heat. I often cover the pan with a lid for a couple of minutes to speed up the cooking. Serve with a dollop of mayo on each side, smoked salmon, red onion and capers in between. You can also add some rocket or spinach leaves.

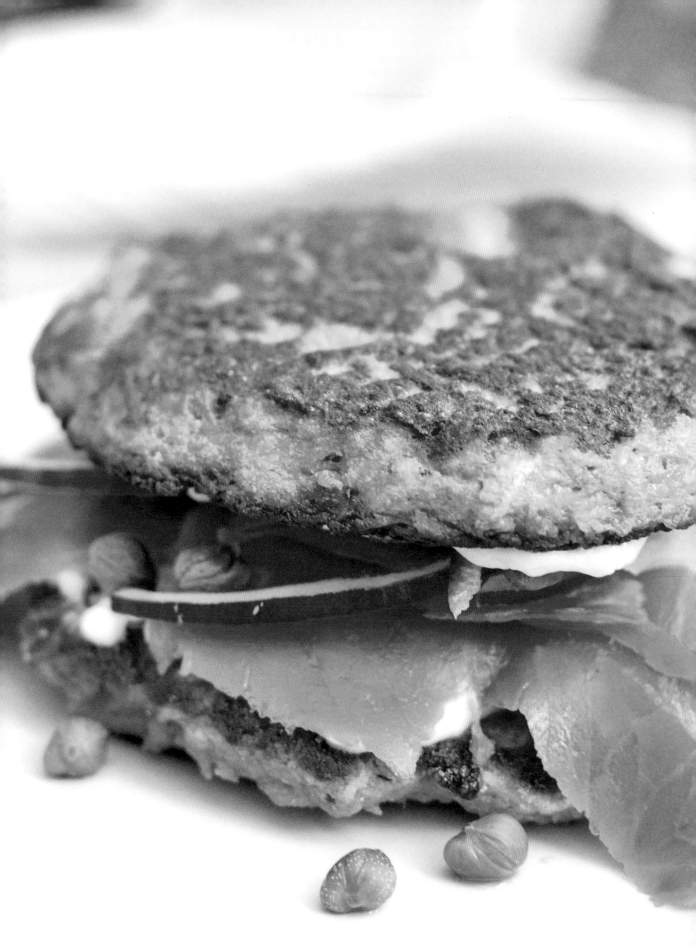

superstar egg muffins

Major disclosure: this is not my recipe! Yes, I've made something similar before but not in this particular combination. It was actually my boyfriend's creation but I have his permission to use it in this cookbook because it's a favourite at home and everyone absolutely loves these easy, tasty muffins.

SERVES 3

1–2 tbsp virgin olive oil

1 small brown onion, diced

4–5 slices of salami or chorizo sausage, diced

4 thick slices of haloumi cheese

6 eggs

Pinch of salt and pepper

Heat virgin olive oil and cook onion until soft and golden, about 4–5 minutes. Remove onion from pan and add salami, cook until browned and crispy. Remove salami and add haloumi cheese, cook until a golden brown crust forms, about a minute on each side. Remove haloumi and cut into small pieces. Set pre-cooked ingredients aside.

Preheat oven to 170°C (335°F). Spray muffin casings with some olive oil.

Whisk eggs with a pinch of salt and pepper. Divide precooked ingredients between muffin casings, about a tablespoon each. Make sure you have an even amount of all three ingredients. Divide and pour the egg mix on top. Carefully transfer the muffin tray to oven and bake for 17 minutes or until the egg muffins have risen and firmed up.

The muffins will drop but stay in shape once you remove them from the oven. We eat these with a side of avocado, cherry tomatoes, sauerkraut and chilli sauce.

Haloumi cheese is a salty, semi-hard cheese, traditionally made with goat and/or sheep's milk, and sometimes with an addition of cow's milk. We pre-cook haloumi cheese, onion and salami the night before to save time in the morning. You can omit haloumi cheese and use other combinations such as sun-dried tomatoes and mushrooms or pre-cooked spinach.

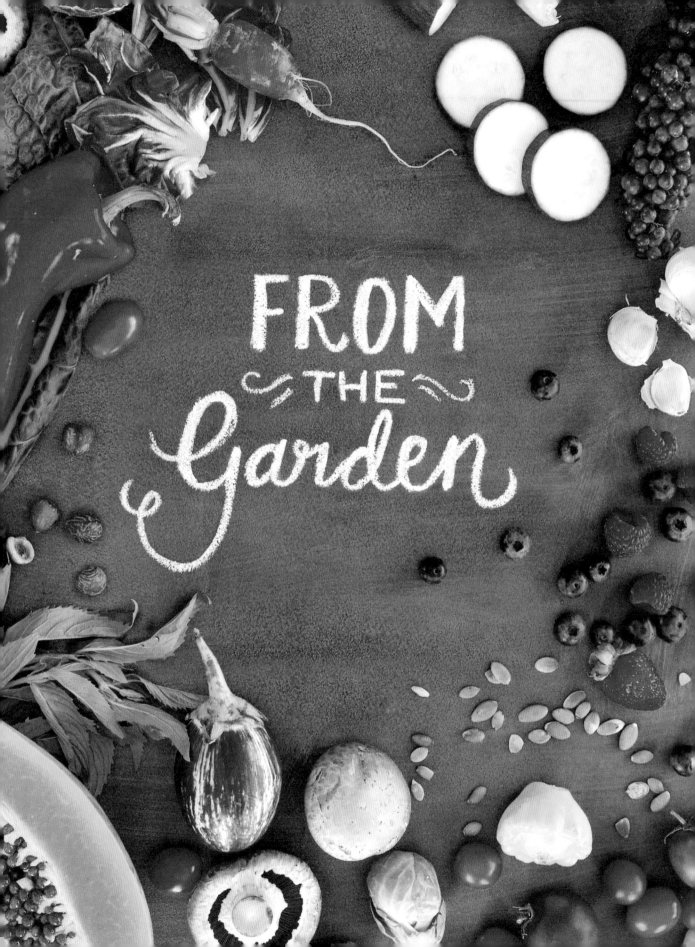

FROM THE Garden

asparagus with warm mushroom dressing

SERVES 2–3

60ml virgin olive oil or macadamia oil

1/2 brown onion, diced

15g dried porcini mushrooms, soaked

7 button mushrooms, diced

1 garlic clove, chopped

1 tbsp verjuice or white wine vinegar

2/3 tsp sea salt

1/2 tsp ground black pepper

1 tsp coconut oil or ghee

2 bunches of green asparagus, ends chopped off

Drizzle of truffle oil (optional) and fresh parsley to serve

Heat olive oil to medium in a frying pan.
Add onion and sauté for 5 minutes, until soft.
Chop rehydrated porcini mushrooms and button mushrooms and cook for a further 3–4 minutes.
Add garlic, verjuice or vinegar, salt and pepper.
Cook for a further few minutes and set aside.

Heat ghee or coconut oil in a frying pan. Add asparagus spears and cook for a minute on each side, just to get a few grill marks. Arrange on a platter and cover with the warm mushroom dressing. Drizzle with truffle oil and scatter with chopped parsley before serving.

You can use the same mushroom dressing on other grilled vegetables or serve it on top of chicken or steaks. Dried porcini mushrooms can be purchased from most fresh food stores. Use leftover dried porcini in a sweet potato shepherd's pie, in a mushroom soup and sauces.

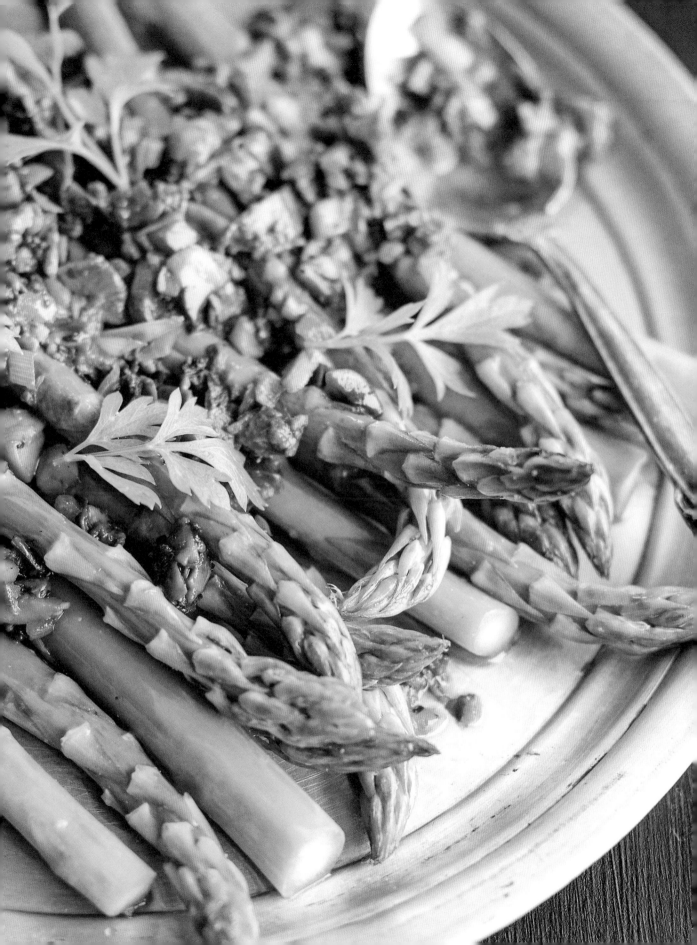

lemongrass pumpkin soup

This is one of the best pumpkin soups I've ever had. No kidding! This is really tasty and really easy to make as long as you have most ingredients on hand.

SERVES 2

1 brown onion, diced

1 lemongrass stalk, cut in thirds

1 long red chilli, diced and deseeded

2 tbsp diced fresh coriander stalks

2cm piece fresh galangal

2cm piece turmeric

4 kaffir lime leaves, optional

2 tsp coconut oil

450g pumpkin, peeled and cubed

1 large garlic clove, chopped

Peel of 1/2 fresh lime

2 tbsp fish sauce

1 litre vegetable stock

100ml coconut cream, plus extra to serve

2 tbsp lime juice

Coriander leaves and sliced chilli to serve

Sauté onion, lemongrass, chilli, coriander stalks, galangal, turmeric and kaffir lime leaves in coconut oil, on medium heat, for 2–3 minutes. Add pumpkin, garlic, lime peel, fish sauce and vegetable stock and bring to boil. Turn the heat down and simmer for 15 minutes, covered with a lid, until pumpkin is soft when poked with a knife.

Remove turmeric, galangal, lime peel, kaffir lime and lemongrass from the soup and transfer the rest to a food processor or a blender. Purée until smooth, in batches if needed, then add coconut cream and lime juice. Whiz a couple more times to incorporate. Serve with a ripple of coconut cream and fresh coriander leaves on top.

Fresh roots can be replaced with 2/3 tsp turmeric powder and 2/3 tsp galangal powder. Butternut squash can be used; sweet potato and carrots would also work well. Coconut milk can be used instead of coconut cream, but put the tin/jar in the fridge for an hour or so to thicken the top half of the liquid.

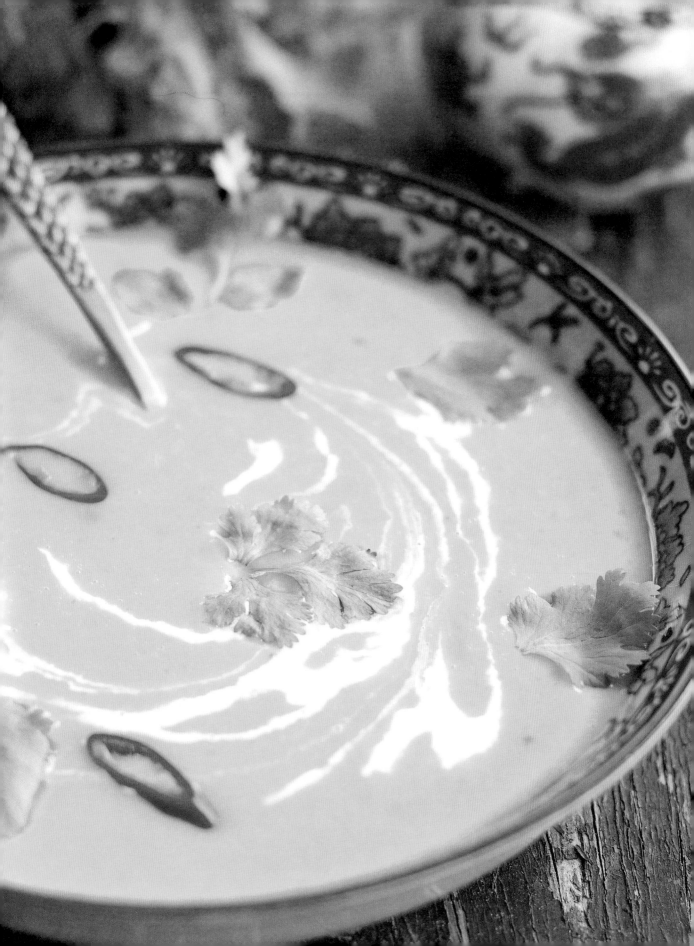

smoked chicken slaw

Both traditional coleslaw and a Ukrainian salad, 'Dnestr', made with the local sliced salami and tinned peas, inspire this salad. It's very versatile – you can make it for lunch or dinner, take it to picnics and barbecues or divide into batches for quick and easy lunches.

SERVES 6

1/2 small cabbage, shredded

2 medium carrots, peeled and grated

2 smoked chicken breasts, sliced

65g green peas (thawed out if frozen)

1 small red onion, finely sliced

2 tbsp finely diced fresh dill

For the dressing

4 tbsp mayonnaise

1 tbsp extra-virgin olive oil

3 tbsp white wine vinegar

2/3 tsp sea salt

2/3 tsp ground black pepper

In a large bowl, mix cabbage, carrots, chicken, peas, onion and fresh dill.

In a separate bowl, whisk the dressing ingredients until well incorporated. Dress the salad 10 minutes before serving to draw out some juices from the cabbage.

Good quality sliced ham or cooked chicken can be used instead of smoked chicken. Try to use a mayonnaise made with olive or macadamia oil, find a recipe on page 187. If you plan to store a batch of salad as leftovers, hold the dressing until you're ready to eat it. This will keep the salad fresh and crispy in the fridge for a few days.

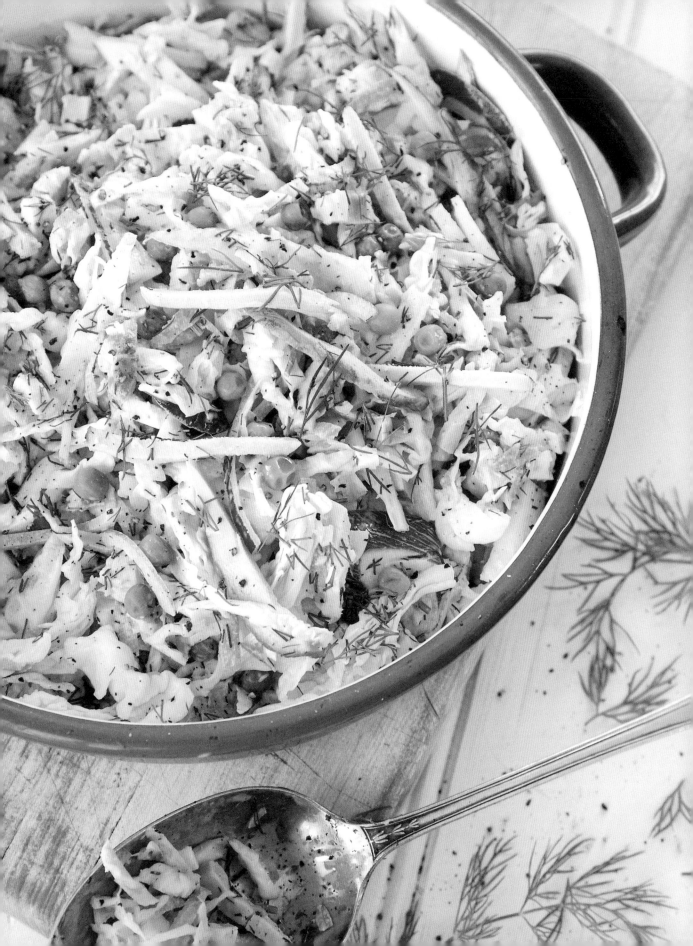

kale avocado gazpacho

Inspired by a traditional tomato gazpacho, this refreshing green soup is like an IV full of antioxidants and healthy fats. Perfect for those days when your body needs a little detox and rejuvenation.

MAKES 2–3 SERVINGS

7–8 kale leaves, washed

1 celery stick with leaves

Juice of 2 limes, zest of 1 for garnish

200ml water

2 spring onions, diced

1 garlic clove, chopped

1/4 cucumber, chopped and peeled

3 tbsp extra-virgin olive oil

1 avocado

2/3 tsp sea salt and black pepper

Handful of fresh parsley or basil

Juice the kale and celery. Grate a teaspoon of lime zest and reserve for later. Add the kale and celery juice and the rest of ingredients to a blender or a food processor, reserving some chopped spring onions and basil for serving

Process until smooth and refrigerate for at least 10 minutes before serving in small bowls or chilled glasses. Garnish with lime zest, fresh basil leaves and some cracked black pepper.

simple roasted pepper gazpacho

SERVES 2

2 red peppers

Dollop of coconut oil

4 medium tomatoes

2 garlic cloves, chopped

1/2 red onion, diced

1 cucumber, peeled and diced

60ml extra-virgin olive oil

325ml cup water

Juice of 1/2 lemon

1 tsp balsamic vinegar

2/3 tsp sea salt and pepper

Preheat oven to 200°C (400°F). Rub the peppers with coconut oil and place on a foil-covered roasting tray. Roast until soft and charred, about 50 minutes, turning after 25 minutes.

In the meantime, bring a saucepan of water to boil and cook tomatoes for 30 seconds. Rinse under cold water, peel the skin off and chop roughly (you can remove the seeds if you like).

Transfer cooked peppers to a plate and, once cooled, remove the skin and the seeds. Place all ingredients in a blender or food processor and puree until smooth. This soup goes nicely with a side of grilled chorizo or prawns.

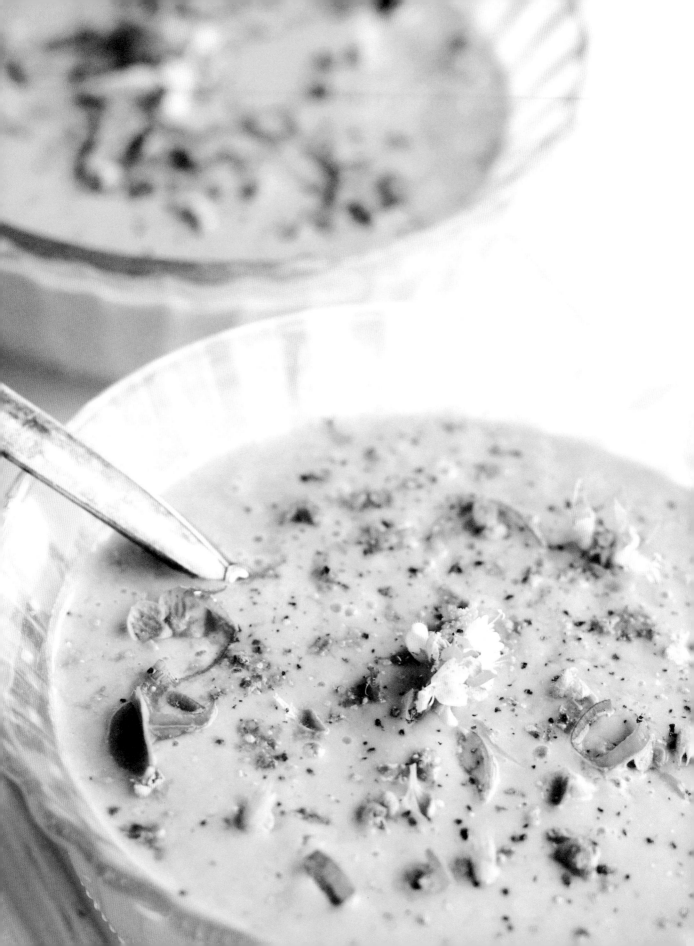

mash three ways

I grew up on mashed potato – eating it with my grandmother's amazing meatballs, marinated tomatoes or with a herring salad. Enjoy these paleo-friendly mushy sides with your favourite roast meat or grilled fish. Use leftovers for a pie crust or as a side with your eggs in the morning. Makes 750ml.

SWEET POTATO BACON MASH

1 large sweet potato, peeled and cut in cubes

2 rashers of bacon, rind removed, diced

1–2 tbsp ghee (butter if you have dairy)

60ml almond milk

2/3 tsp sea salt

1/2 tsp black pepper

1/2 tsp of Dijon mustard

1 tbsp of Parmesan cheese, grated (optional)

Place sweet potato in a medium saucepan of water, bring to boil and cook for about 10–15 minutes, until soft when poked through with a knife. Strain and set aside. Meanwhile, pan-fry bacon pieces in a little ghee until crisp. Remove to a plate and pour the fat from the frying pan into the cooked sweet potato. Add one tablespoon of ghee, almond milk, salt, pepper and mustard. Mash or purée in a food processor until smooth. Add a little cheese if you like. Finally, fold through crispy bacon and sprinkle a few pieces on top.

BROCCOLI & RICOTTA MASH

1 medium white potato, peeled and cubed

1 small head broccoli, broken into florets

2 tbsp ricotta cheese

Zest of 1 lemon

1 tbsp lemon juice

1/2 tsp sea salt

Pinch of black pepper

1 tbsp olive oil

Fresh parsley or mint to serve

Place potato in cold water and bring to boil. Cook for 10 minutes, add broccoli and cook for a further 5 minutes until both vegetables are soft. Strain and place potato and broccoli in a food processor with ricotta cheese, lemon zest, lemon juice, salt, pepper and olive oil. Process until smooth. Garnish with fresh parsley or mint.

Continued on page 62.

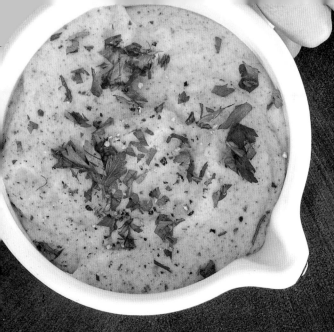

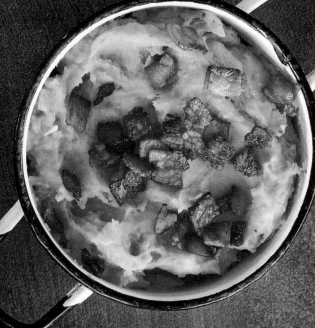

BROCCOLi

SWEET POTATO

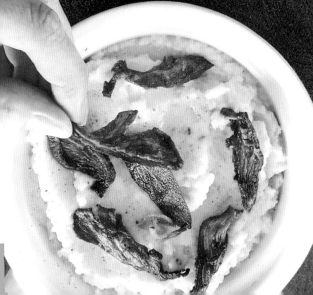

Cauliflower

mash three ways

CAULIFLOWER SAGE BUTTER MASH

1/2 head cauliflower, cut into florets

50g butter

Handful of fresh sage leaves

2 garlic cloves, sliced

2/3 tsp sea salt

125ml almond milk or vegetable stock

Smoked oyster mushrooms (page 164) to serve

Continued from page 60.

Bring a medium saucepan of water to boil and cook cauliflower for 15 minutes until very soft. Strain and place in a food processor.

Meanwhile, melt butter over medium heat and add sage, garlic, and a pinch of salt. Cook until butter foams and turns golden, and the sage leaves turn crispy. Remove sage leaves and add the butter with garlic to cauliflower. Add almond milk or vegetable stock to the food processor and purée everything into smooth mash. Season with a pinch of salt and pepper to taste. Top with crispy sage leaves and smoky oyster mushrooms to serve.

baked parsnips with sage

SERVES 2

10 parsnips, peeled and cut in halves

3 tbsp ghee, melted

15 fresh sage leaves

Peel of 1 lemon, in strips

3 garlic cloves

Pinch of salt

2 tbsp lemon juice

Preheat oven to 180°C (355°F). Toss parsnips in melted ghee and roast for 10 minutes. Add sage leaves, lemon peel, lemon juice and garlic and roast for a further 15 minutes. Sprinkle with salt and drizzle with extra lemon juice before serving.

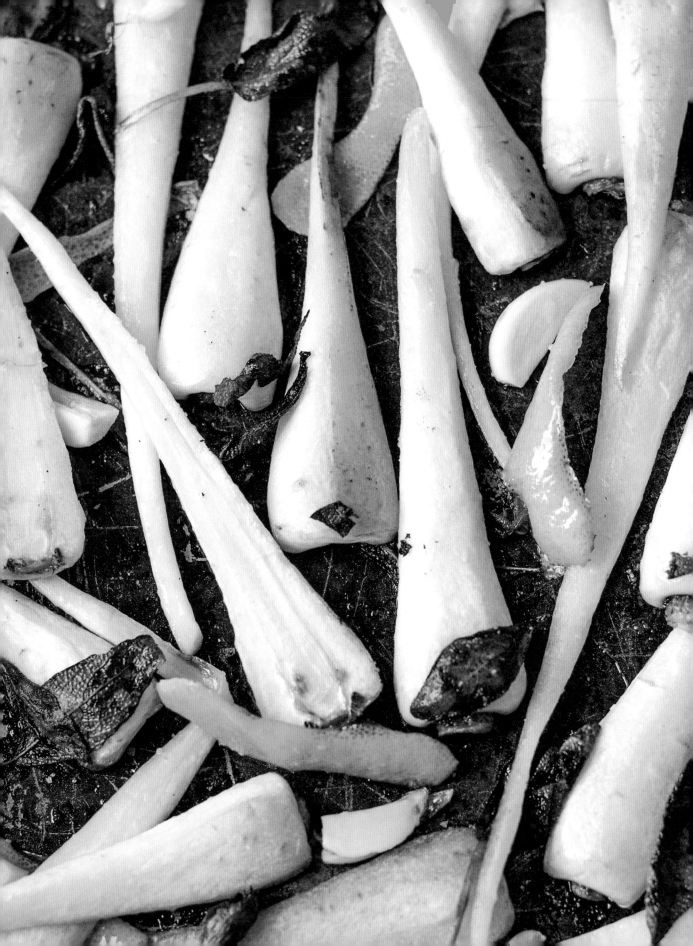

cauliflower steaks with braised radicchio

SERVES 2

1 tsp coconut oil

1 medium cauliflower head, cut into 1–2cm thick steaks

Pinch of sea salt and ground black pepper

For radicchio

1 tbsp ghee

3–4 shallots, sliced

2 garlic cloves, chopped

2/3 tsp sea salt

1/2 tsp ground black pepper

2 tbsp verjuice or 1 tbsp white wine vinegar

1/2 radicchio, shredded

Handful of watercress or baby spinach

1 tbsp extra-virgin olive oil

Squeeze of lemon juice

Preheat oven to 200°C (390°F). Heat coconut oil in a frying pan until sizzling hot. Add cauliflower steaks and fry for 2 minutes on each side, until golden brown. Sprinkle with a pinch of salt and pepper and transfer to a roasting tray. Bake in the oven for 15 minutes.

Meanwhile, heat 1 tablespoon of ghee in a frying pan and sauté sliced shallots for 5 minutes on medium heat. Add garlic, salt, pepper, and verjuice and cook for a further 2–3 minutes. Add shredded radicchio, stir through and cook for 1–2 minutes, until slightly wilted.

Serve cauliflower steaks topped with braised radicchio and watercress or spinach drizzled with olive oil, and lemon juice on the side.

Use leftover cauliflower florets for roasting, see recipe on page 162, or in cauliflower fritters.

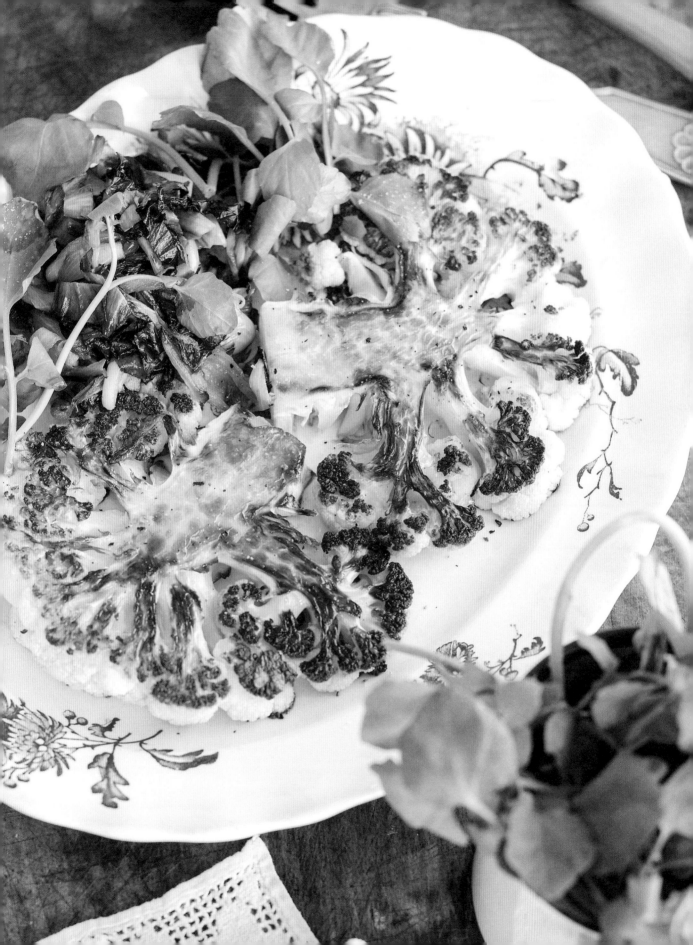

courgette carbonara

Contrary to the popular belief that the creaminess of a carbonara comes from cream, it's actually the lightly cooked eggs that coat the pasta, together with some melted Parmesan cheese. Using courgette instead of pasta creates a guilt-free version of the classic and lemon zest adds a little freshness.

SERVES 2

1 tsp ghee or macadamia oil

4 rashers of bacon, diced

1 tbsp virgin olive oil

1 garlic clove, finely chopped

4 courgettes, sliced into thin strips

1 tsp grated lemon zest

1/2 tsp sea salt

2/3 tsp ground black pepper

2 eggs

2 tbsp grated Parmesan cheese

Heat ghee in a frying pan until sizzling hot. Add bacon and fry until crispy all over.

Turn the heat to medium. Add olive oil and garlic and cook for a couple of minutes. Add courgettes, lemon zest, salt and pepper and stir through. Cook briefly, for about a minute, before adding 2 whole eggs. Keep stirring until the courgettes are well coated and the egg starts to cook and thicken, it should only take about a minute or two. Don't overcook the courgettes as it's all about the crunch. Finally, turn the heat off and fold in the Parmesan cheese.

Those avoiding all dairy can use a couple of tablepsoons of nutritional yeast instead of Parmesan cheese.

asian sesame cucumber salad

SERVES 4

4–5 shitake mushrooms, sliced

1 tsp ghee

4 Lebanese cucumbers, thinly shaved or sliced

2 tbsp white or black sesame seeds

For the dressing

1 tsp sesame oil

2 tbsp extra-virgin olive oil

1 tsp fish sauce

2 tbsp lime juice

1 tbsp coconut aminos

Pan-fry sliced shitake mushrooms in ghee over medium heat for 3–4 minutes, until lightly browned on each side. Remove to a bowl with sliced cucumbers. Whisk together the dressing and combine with cucumbers and mushrooms. Toss with sesame seeds, which you can lightly toast beforehand.

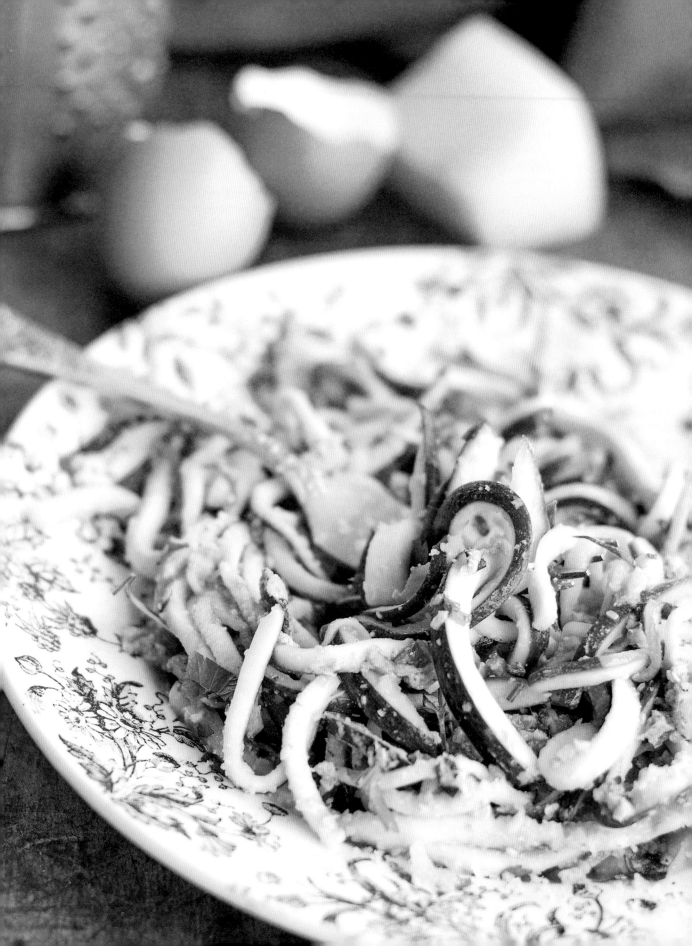

cavolo nero

Cavolo nero is another green leafy vegetable to add to your cooking repertoire. It has narrow, wrinkled, dark green leaves and a mild flavour, similar to kale. It's great in soups and salads but I love it sautéed and combined with punchy flavours.

SERVES 2

2 garlic cloves, roughly diced

30g macadamia nuts

8–10 sun-dried tomatoes, roughly diced

1 tbsp grated lemon zest

4 tbsp virgin olive oil

Bunch of cavolo nero (8 leaves), chopped

125ml verjuice or white wine

2/3 tsp sea salt

Pinch of ground black pepper

1 tbsp butter (ghee if avoiding dairy)

Juice of 1/4 lemon

In a food processor, grind garlic, macadamia nuts, sun-dried tomatoes, lemon zest and 2 tbsp of olive oil into a crumbly mixture.

Heat 2 tbsp of olive oil in a large frying pan. Add the nut mixture and sauté for 3–4 minutes until fragrant and the garlic is slightly golden brown. Add cavolo nero and verjuice and sauté together for 5 minutes on medium heat. Add salt, pepper and butter and cook for a further 5 minutes. Drizzle with some lemon juice just before serving.

This dish can be served with eggs for breakfast or with fish or meat for lunch and dinner. Similar to kale, cavolo nero can also be made into chips or juiced to make green power smoothies.

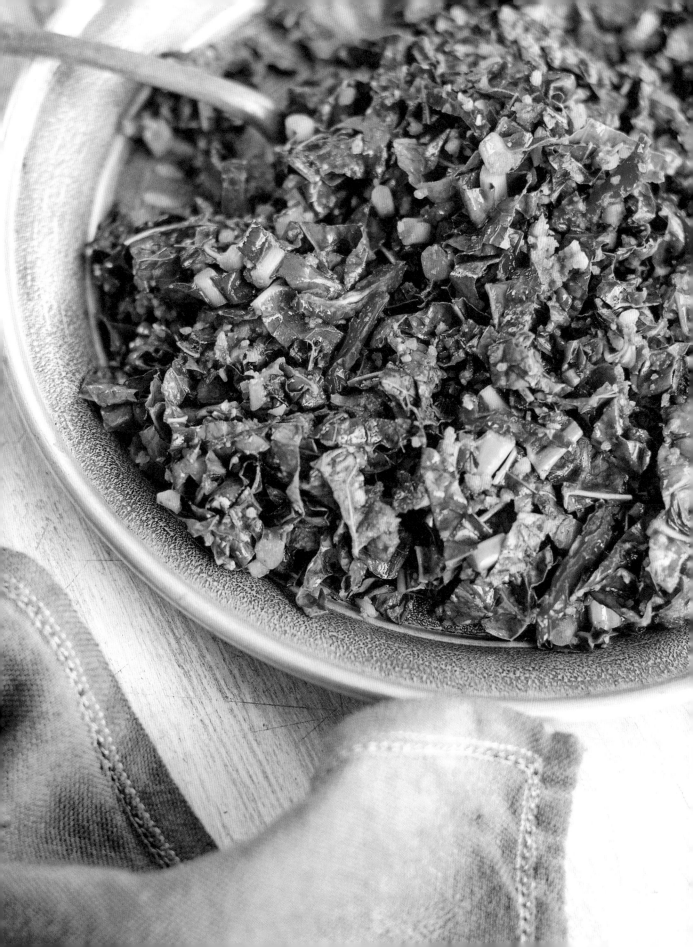

ratatouille cake

Well before it was made famous by a certain Pixar rat, a hearty ratatouille was a regular vegetable dish at our home. This particular recipe is a ratatouille on steroids – even more vegetable goodness and flavour packed into a grandiose-looking layered cake.

SERVES 8

3 large aubergines, sliced lengthways, 1cm thick

1–2 tsp sea salt

2 large courgettes, sliced lengthways, 5mm thick

2 red peppers, sliced into long strips

4 tbsp virgin olive oil

3 tbsp tomato purée

2 tbsp fresh thyme leaves

2 garlic cloves, finely chopped

Sea salt and pepper

It helps to sprinkle aubergine slices with salt and set aside for 15 minutes before cooking to draw out some of the juices. Rinse and pat dry with a paper towel before frying. This dish is as good oven-hot as it is cold straight out of the fridge. It will keep for 3–4 days in the refrigerator.

Layer by layer, brush aubergine slices with olive oil. Grill on a hot barbecue, with the lid on, or in a griddle pan for 2–3 minutes on each side, until brown chargrill marks appear and the aubergine softens. Toss courgette and red pepper slices in olive oil and a few pinches of salt and barbecue or griddle for a few minutes on each side.

Preheat oven to 200°C (390°F). Line a 20cm cake tin with foil – this will prevent any leakage. Line the foil with baking paper. Cover the bottom and sides of the tin with a single layer of overlapping aubergine slices, avoid any gaps. Spread half of the tomato purée on the first layer of aubergine, sprinkle with a third of fresh thyme leaves, a third of the garlic and a pinch of salt and ground black pepper. Add a layer of red peppers, covering as much of the bottom and sides as possible. Follow with a layer of courgette and sprinkle another third of thyme and garlic. Now, add another layer of aubergine followed by the remaining tomato purée, thyme and garlic, and another pinch of salt and pepper. Fill in the middle with the remaining aubergine. Press everything down, making sure the whole surface is covered. Bake in the oven for 20 minutes.

Cool down to room temperature, for about 1 hour. Place a serving plate, face down, on top of the vegetable cake. Pressing the plate down, carefully turn the tin upside down. Once it feels securely on the plate, remove the tin, foil and paper. Some of the juices will leak out but the cake should hold shape even when you cut it. Garnish with a few sprigs of thyme.

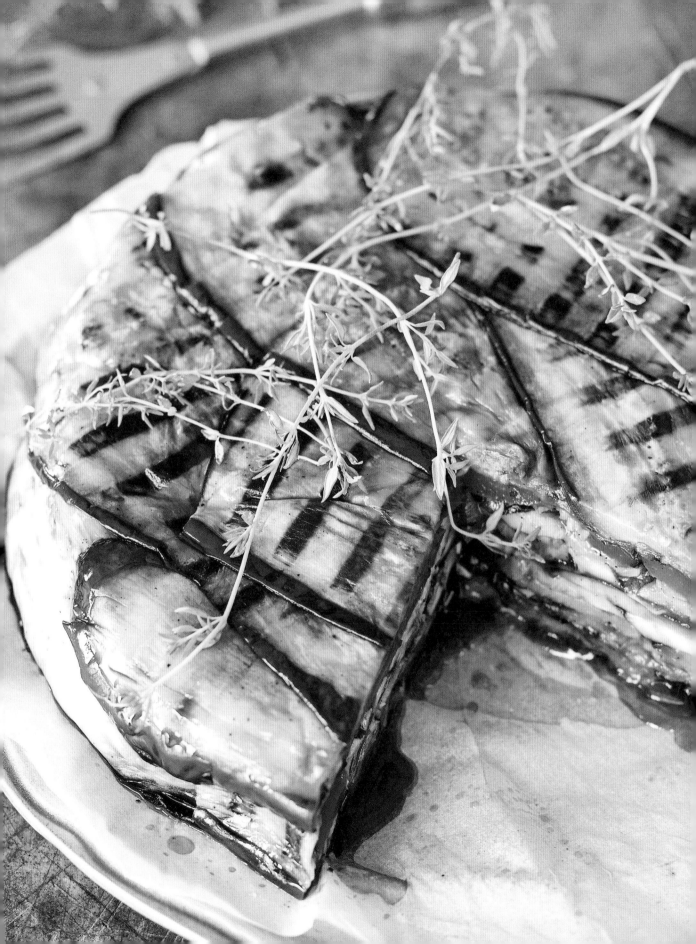

roasted brussels sprouts

SERVES 4

500g brussels sprouts, washed
and halved

150g sliced speck or bacon

1–2 tbsp macadamia or coconut oil

2 tbsp extra-virgin olive oil

1 tbsp vino cotto or sweet
balsamic vinegar

1/2 tsp hot mustard

Juice of 1/2 lime

1/2 tsp grated garlic

1 tsp sea salt

1/2 tsp ground black pepper

10 cherry tomatoes, halved

Preheat oven to 200°C (390°F). Toss brussels sprouts and speck slices in macadamia or coconut oil and roast for 30 minutes, until crisped and browned. Stir halfway through roasting.

Whisk together olive oil, vino cotto, mustard, lime juice, garlic, salt and pepper. Add fresh cherry tomatoes to roasted brussels sprouts and speck and toss together with the dressing. Serve in the same roasting tray or in a salad bowl.

> Speck is similar to prosciutto and other smoked hams made from the pig's shoulder. Make your own hot mustard from page 200. Vino cotto is a naturally sweet 'cooked wine' syrup, similar to caramelised balsamic vinegar but not as sour. Sweet balsamic can also be used, or you can add a little honey to regular balsamic vinegar instead.

brussels sprouts with cranberries

SERVES 2

2 tbsp macadamia oil or ghee

1 medium brown onion, thinly sliced

About 15–20 brussels sprouts, sliced

2 garlic cloves, finely chopped

2/3 tsp salt

1 tsp ghee or butter

Generous pinch of pepper

1 tsp balsamic vinegar

25g dried cranberries

Heat oil or ghee in a frying pan and sauté onion until soft and translucent.

In the meantime, shred the brussels sprouts. Cut the ends off the sprouts and slice them in half lengthways. Then slice each half into thin strips. Add to the onion together with garlic, salt and butter. Cook for 2–3 minutes, stirring occasionally, and then add the pepper, balsamic vinegar and cranberries. Stir through and cook for a further 2–3 minutes.

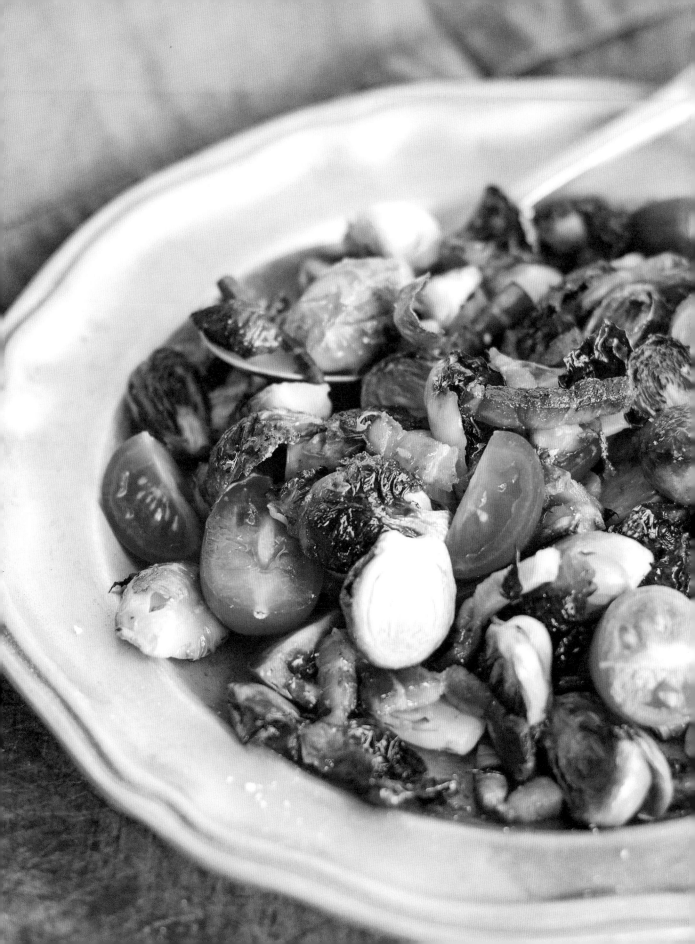

cauliflower couscous

I make cauliflower couscous whenever I serve a hearty meat or fish tagine or some Moroccan spiced lamb cutlets. It's really fast and easy to prepare but make sure not to overcook the cauliflower or it will lose its crunch. You can use a variety of spice mixes for seasoning.

SERVES 3-4

1 head of cauliflower, broken into florets

2 tbsp ghee

1 brown onion, finely diced

60g raw pistachio nuts

2 garlic cloves, finely chopped

Zest from 1 small lemon

1 tsp sea salt

1/2 tsp black pepper

2/3 tsp turmeric powder

2/3 tsp curry powder

Juice from 1/2 lemon

3 tbsp extra-virgin olive oil

Handful of fresh parsley, chopped

40g pomegranate seeds

Extra nuts for garnish

Place cauliflower into a food processor and grind into small crumbs. You can use your knife skills but the crumbs might not end up as small. Set aside in a bowl.

Heat 1 tablespoon of ghee in a large frying pan on medium. Sauté diced onion for 7–8 minutes until soft. Meanwhile, grind pistachio nuts into small crumbs in a food processor or with a mortar and pestle.

Add processed nuts, garlic, lemon zest and another tablespoon of ghee to the frying pan and stir for a minute or two. Then add the salt, pepper, turmeric and curry powder and stir for another minute. Finally add the cauliflower, mix through really well and cook for 1 to 2 minutes. Drizzle with lemon juice and olive oil and add chopped parsley and pomegranate seeds. Combine and serve with extra pistachio nuts on top.

Pomegranate can be replaced with diced dried fruit such as apricots, figs or cranberries. Other nuts can be used instead of pistachios.

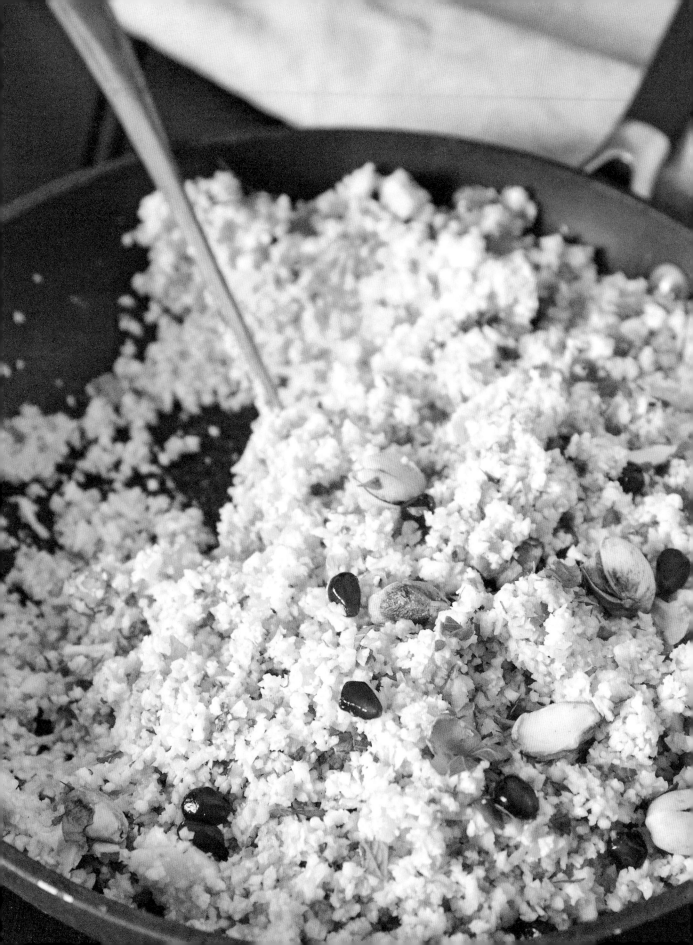

dukkah-spiced roasted squash

Squash and dukkah spices go really well together. This is a quick and easy way of pairing them up but you could alternatively toss the squash in coconut oil and coat in dukkah before roasting in the oven. Sun-dried tomatoes add acidity and pumpkin seeds add a little crunch to the dish. Make extra to pack for lunch the next day.

SERVES 3

1/2 small winter squash

1 tbsp coconut oil

2 tbsp dukkah spice mix

2/3 tsp sea salt

25g sun-dried tomatoes, sliced

1 tbsp pumpkin seeds

Preheat oven to 200°C (390°F). Cut squash into 1cm slices, remove seeds and toss with melted coconut oil (macadamia oil or ghee can also be used). Roast on a flat baking tray for 25–30 minutes. Serve sprinkled with dukkah spice mix, salt, sun-dried tomatoes and pumpkin seeds.

You can buy dukkah spice mix in most supermarkets and delis or make your own.

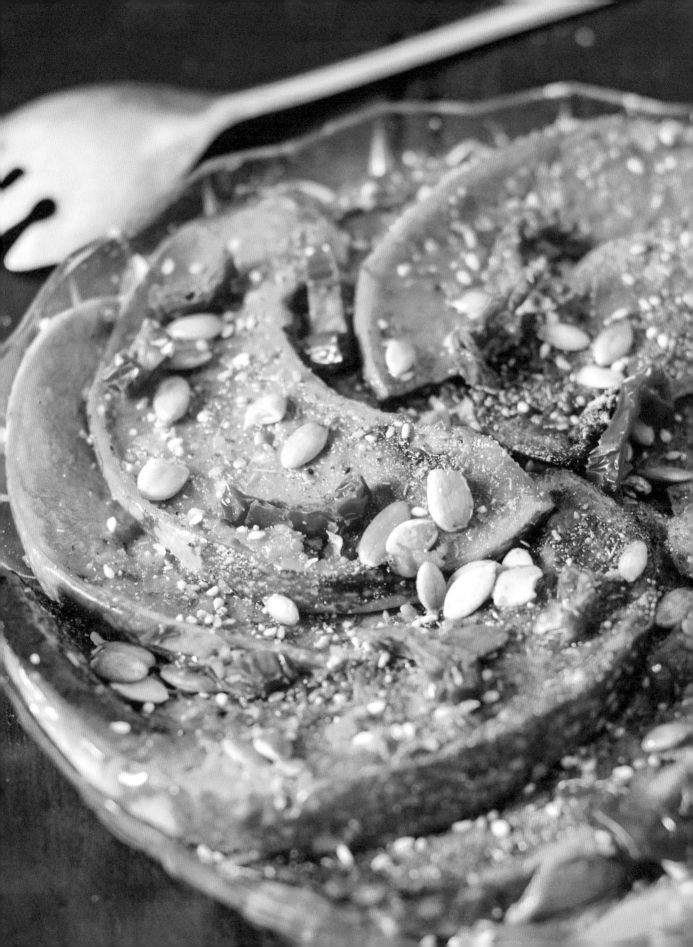

nectarine & quail egg salad

Just by adding quail eggs and some fresh, sweet nectarine you can transform a simple garden salad into a fancy looking dish. Free-range chicken eggs can easily be used instead.

SERVES 2

10 quail eggs

5 tbsp extra-virgin olive oil

2 tbsp white wine vinegar

Pinch of salt

Pinch of ground black pepper

2/3 tsp Dijon mustard

10 basil leaves

50g rocket, washed

1/2 red pepper, sliced

10 cherry tomatoes, halved

1/2 red onion, thinly sliced

1–2 nectarines, sliced

1 tsp black sesame seeds

Remove quail eggs from the fridge half an hour before cooking. Bring a medium saucepan of water to boil, gently immerse eggs and cook for 5 minutes. Rinse under cold water, peel and cut in half.

Using a food processor or a blender, purée and blend olive oil, vinegar, salt, pepper, mustard and basil leaves into a dressing.

Mix rocket with red pepper slices, cherry tomatoes and onion and assemble on a platter. Top with quail eggs and nectarine slices and drizzle with the basil dressing. Sprinkle with a little sea salt and black sesame seeds.

You can use white sesame seeds instead. Peaches can be used instead of nectarines and regular eggs can be cooked instead of quail eggs.

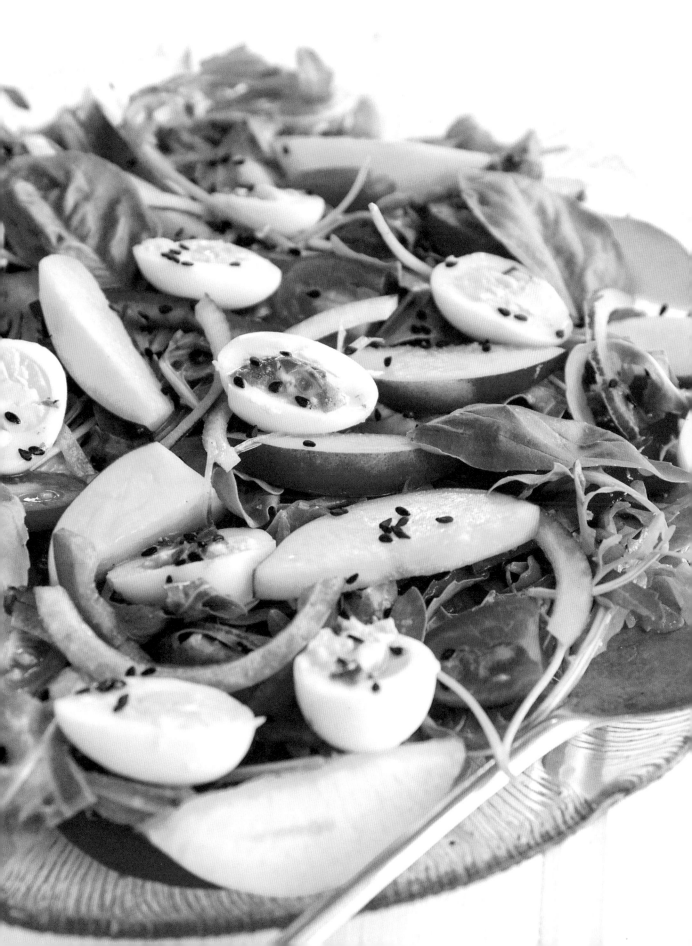

ruby grapefruit & fennel salad

I make this salad when people come over for dinner because it looks so pretty and fresh on the table. Crispy, tangy and bursting with flavour, it will brighten up any winter dinner and cool you off on a hot summer's day. Pro tip: it goes really well with lamb cutlets.

SERVES 2

1 pink grapefruit

1/2 fennel bulb, thinly sliced or shaved

1 avocado, sliced

1/4 red onion, finely sliced

60g mixed green salad, shredded

For the dressing

1 tsp grapefruit zest

1 tsp lemon zest

2 tbsp lemon juice

2 tbsp extra-virgin olive oil

1 tsp mayonnaise

2/3 tsp raw honey or maple syrup

Pinch of sea salt and pepper

A few mint leaves and fennel fronds (green tips)

Grate some of the zest before cutting off the base and top of the grapefruit and sitting it flat on your cutting board. Slice the sides to remove the skin and white pith. Holding the grapefruit over a bowl to catch any juice, cut it into segments. Pour the juice into a separate bowl and mix with the rest of the dressing ingredients.

Combine grapefruit, fennel, avocado, onion and salad leaves with the dressing and top with a few mint leaves and fennel fronds.

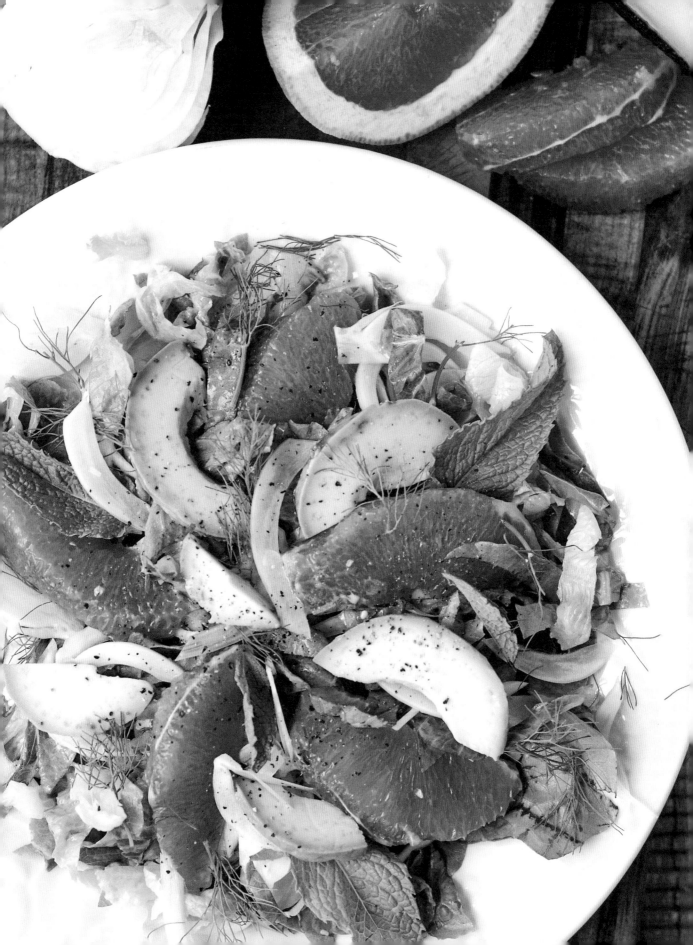

sage and pancetta sweet potato

Burnt butter sauce is a favourite of mine but you can use ghee – clarified butter – if you're avoiding dairy as it's 95 per cent fat with practically no milk solids. Olive oil could also be used but you'd be missing out on the gorgeous nutty flavour of burnt butter.

SERVES 2

1 medium sweet potato, halved lengthways

2 tbsp virgin olive oil

4–6 slices of pancetta

2 tbsp butter or ghee

2/3 tsp sea salt

1/2 tsp ground black pepper

Pinch of ground nutmeg

2 garlic cloves, sliced

20–25 fresh sage leaves

Preheat oven to 200°C (390°F). Place sweet potato halves on a baking paper-lined tray, flesh-side up, and bake for 35–40 minutes until very soft and the skin is browned.

Meanwhile, heat a tablespoon of olive oil in a frying pan and cook pancetta slices for a couple of minutes on each side until crispy. Remove to a side plate and reserve the cooking fats.

Five minutes before the sweet potatoes are ready, place the frying pan back on medium heat. Add another tablespoon of olive oil and 2 tablespoons of butter and wait until melted. Add salt, pepper, nutmeg, garlic slices and sage leaves and cook until the butter foams, the garlic browns slightly and the sage leaves turn crispy – around 3–5 minutes.

Serve sweet potato halves drizzled with butter sauce, sage leaves and garlic with crispy pancetta on the side.

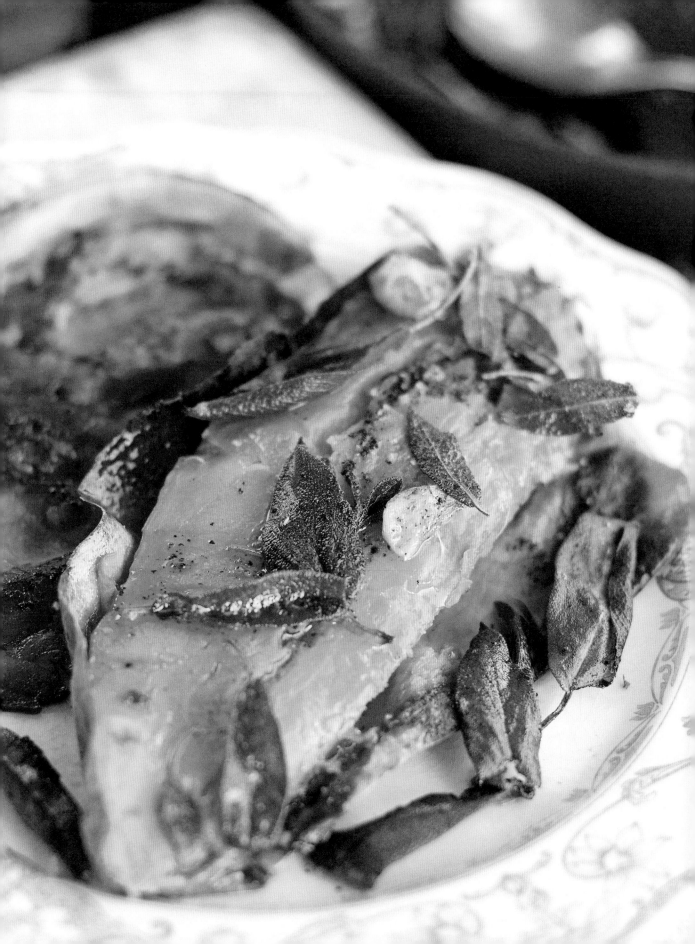

moroccan aubergine salad

Aubergine is one my favourite vegetables to cook with – I love its smoky, almost meaty flavour and silky, soft texture. It's particularly tasty with Middle Eastern spices, garlic and lemon, which form the basis of this salad.

SERVES 4-6

2 large aubergines

2 tsp sea salt

2–3 tbsp coconut oil

2 tsp ghee

1 tbsp virgin olive oil, plus extra to drizzle

1 red pepper, sliced

2 garlic cloves, roughly chopped

1 tsp ground cumin

1/2 tsp coriander seed powder

1/2 tsp chilli powder or chilli flakes

Zest and juice of 1 lemon

4 Roma tomatoes, quartered, seeds removed, then diced

1 red onion, finely sliced

Handful of fresh parsley, chopped

Slice aubergines into discs of 1cm thickness and sprinkle liberally with salt. Set aside for 10 minutes to draw out some of the juices. This will prevent them from soaking up too much oil during cooking. Rinse with cold water and dry with paper towel.

Heat 2 tbsp of coconut oil and one tbsp of ghee in a large frying pan to sizzling hot, make sure the oil is very hot before adding the aubergine to prevent excess absorption. Fry aubergine in batches, for 2–3 minutes on each side, until dark golden brown but not black, as this will make it bitter. Remove to a bowl.

Bring the heat down and add a tablespoon of olive oil to the same frying pan. Add red pepper slices and sauté for a few minutes. Add garlic, cumin, ground coriander seeds, chilli and zest of half a lemon. Cook for a minute or two and add to the bowl with the aubergines. Add tomatoes and red onion. Toss with with lemon juice and a little extra olive oil, and sprinkle with parsley. Season with a little extra sea salt if needed.

Make sure the aubergine is well fried, as that's what gives this dish real depth and smoky flavour. Goes really well with grilled chicken or lamb.

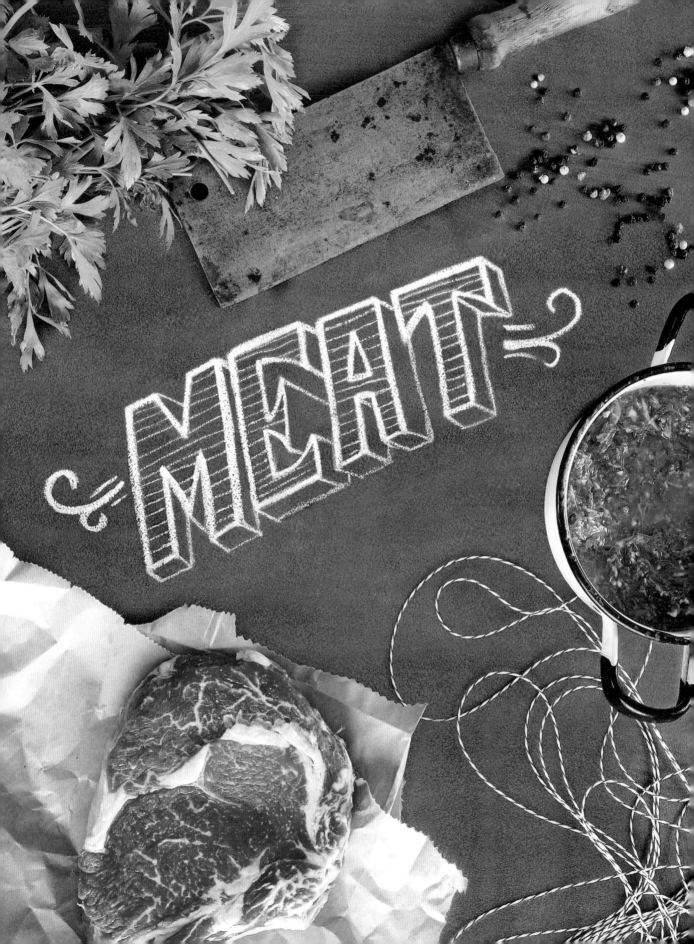

& MEAT

roasted rib-eye with rocket chimichurri

This recipe is designed for two so be prepared to share this chunky, juicy rib-eye. Chimichurri can be made with spinach or other dark green salad leaf instead of rocket. Reserve leftover chimichurri in an airtight container, it will keep for 2–3 days in the fridge.

SERVES 2

500–600g rib-eye steak, 2cm thick on the bone

olive oil

2/3 tsp sea salt

2/3 tsp pepper

1 tsp ghee

For rocket chimichurri

125ml extra-virgin olive oil

2 tbsp white wine vinegar

10g chopped rocket

30g chopped fresh parsley

1 tsp grated lemon zest

1/2 long red chilli, chopped

2 garlic cloves, chopped

1/2 tsp sea salt

Brush the steak with olive oil and season with salt and pepper. Leave on the counter for 20 minutes to bring to room temperature.

Preheat the oven to 170°C (335°F) and heat a grill pan to a high heat. Add ghee and once sizzling, add the steak and cook for 3–4 minutes on each side, until dark brown and sealed. Turn it around with tongs to make sure all sides are browned. Place in an oven tray and roast for 15 minutes for medium rare. Remove and rest the steak on a board covered with foil for 7–8 minutes before slicing.

Meanwhile, place all chimichurri ingredients in a food processor and process until everything is well ground and blended.

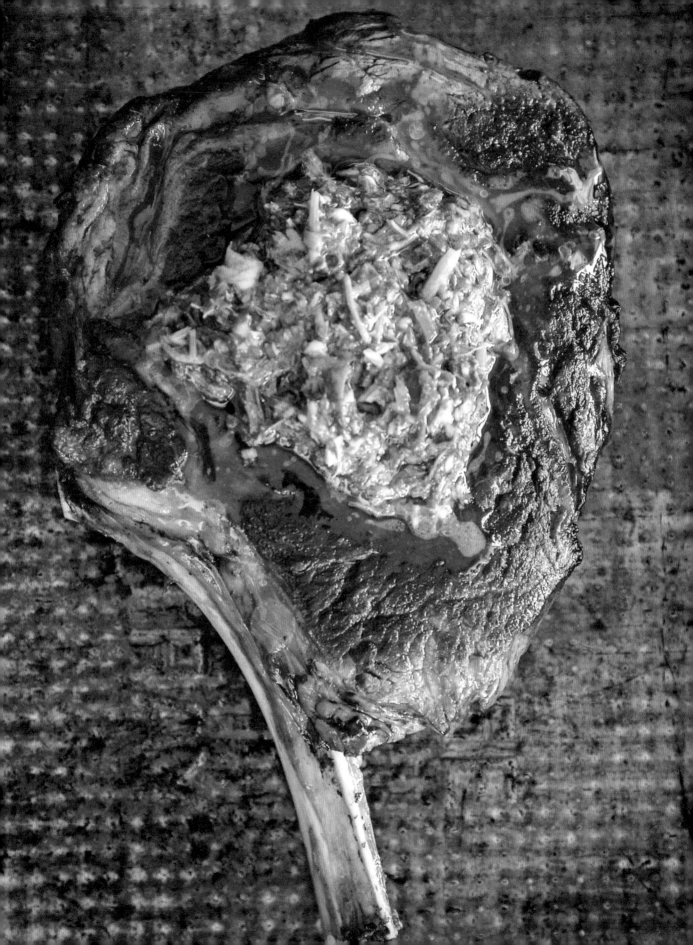

chicken, leek purée & macadamia morsels

This is one of my favourite dishes to make for guests. They're always pleasantly startled by a contrast of flavours and textures – velvety, almost sweet leek purée; savoury, subtly salty chicken; and zesty, crunchy macadamia crumbs. Be a Michelin-starred chef in your own kitchen.

SERVES 3

For chicken

2 chicken breasts, sliced lengthways

1 tbsp Dijon mustard

2/3 tsp sea salt

1 tsp garlic powder

1 tbsp virgin olive oil

1 tsp coconut oil for frying

For leek purée

3 tbsp ghee

2 leeks, sliced (pale and light green part only)

1 potato, peeled and cubed

60ml white wine

1 tsp sea salt

180ml vegetable stock

For macadamia crumbs

65g macadamia nuts

Zest of 1 lemon

1 garlic clove

2 tbsp macadamia or virgin olive oil

1/2 tsp sea salt

2 tbsp lemon juice

1 tbsp fresh oregano leaves

Coat the chicken breast slices with a mix of Dijon mustard, sea salt, garlic powder and virgin olive oil in a bowl. Set aside to marinate for 20 minutes.

For the purée, heat 3 tbsp of ghee in a medium saucepan and sauté the leeks for 10 minutes. Add potato, white wine, salt and vegetable stock, and bring to boil. Turn the heat to medium and cook uncovered for 15 minutes until potato is soft. Transfer to a food processor or a blender and purée until smooth. Return to the saucepan to reheat just before serving.

Place macadamia nuts, lemon zest and garlic in a food processor and grind into small crumbs. Heat the oil in a frying pan to medium and add macadamia mixture and salt. Pan-fry for 3–4 minutes, stirring every 10–15 seconds, until the nuts and garlic start to brown slightly. Turn the heat off, add the lemon juice and stir. Transfer to a bowl.

Heat coconut oil in a frying pan until sizzling hot and turn the heat to medium. Add marinated chicken slices and cook for 5 minutes on each side. Set aside to rest for 2–3 minutes.

Serve chicken breast slices on top of leek purée, sprinkled with a couple of teaspoons of macadamia crumbs and oregano leaves.

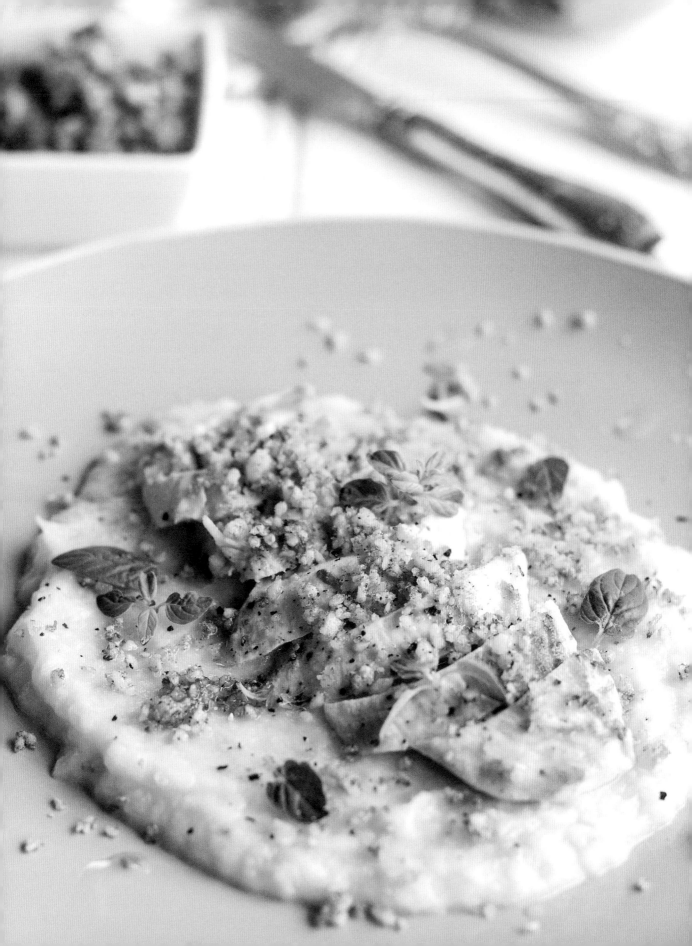

chicken and wild mushroom stew

In this stew the chicken is cooked until very tender and the mushrooms infuse the stew through and through. It's a perfect, hearty dish to share at the family dinner table.

SERVES 4

30g dried wild mushrooms

1 tbsp ghee or coconut oil

1 brown onion, sliced

75g diced speck or bacon

1 celery stick, diced

2 1/2 small chicken breasts, diced

125ml white wine

3 garlic cloves, chopped

500ml chicken stock

125ml soaked mushroom water
(reserved from soaked mushrooms)

3 bay leaves

Pinch of nutmeg

2/3 tsp sea salt

1/2 tsp ground black pepper

2 medium carrots, sliced

6–7 brown mushrooms, sliced

1 medium courgette, sliced

1 tbsp arrowroot powder

1 tsp grated lemon zest to serve

2 tbsp fresh parsley leaves to serve

Soak dry mushrooms in a cup of boiling hot water for 10 minutes.

Heat ghee to medium and sauté onion for 5 minutes. Add speck and celery and cook for a further 3–4 minutes on medium heat. Add diced chicken and cook together for 5 minutes, until the meat is slightly browned.

Add wild mushrooms (reserving the soaking water) and wine and bring the heat up to let it bubble away for a minute. Add garlic, chicken stock, the water from soaked mushrooms, bay leaves, nutmeg, sea salt and pepper. Bring to simmer and cook covered for 40 minutes.

After 40 minutes, add carrots and fresh sliced mushrooms. Cook covered for a further hour, then add courgette and arrowroot powder dissolved in a little water or some of the liquid from the stew. Stir and cook for a further 10 minutes uncovered, until thickened. Sprinkle with lemon zest and fresh parsley before serving.

> Serve with steamed cauliflower, broccoli or green beans. For a slightly higher carbohydrate meal, serve with a side of sweet potato or pumpkin.
>
> Tapioca flour can be used instead of arrowroot.

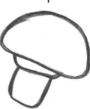

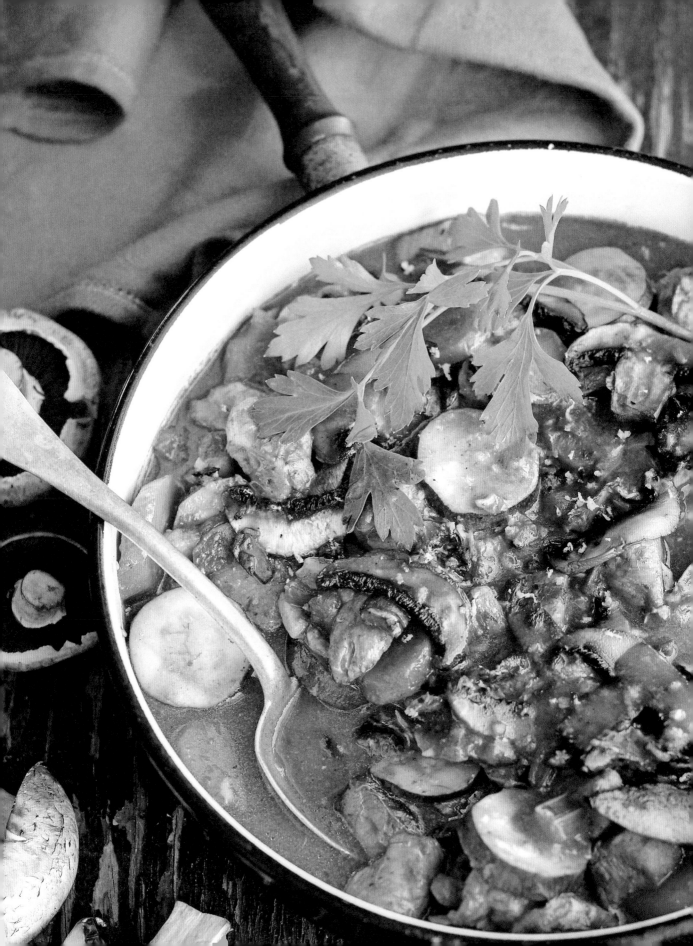

braised cabbage rolls

This dish is an adaptation of traditional Ukrainian cabbage rolls made with minced meat, rice and vegetables. It was one of my favourite family meals growing up. It takes a little effort to prepare the rolls but they keep well in the fridge for the next few days and are totally worth the effort.

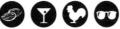

MAKES 12 ROLLS

1 large white cabbage

For the filling

250g pork mince

250g beef mince

55g hazelnut or almond meal

3 garlic cloves, finely chopped

1 onion, finely diced

2 tbsp diced fresh parsley

2 tsp sweet paprika

1 1/2 tsp sea salt

1 tsp mustard (Dijon or wholegrain)

1/2 tsp ground black pepper

1/2 tsp red chilli flakes

2 tbsp pine nuts

2 tbsp virgin olive oil

1 tbsp gluten-free Worcestershire sauce

1 egg

For tomato broth

600g diced tomatoes

1 tsp tomato purée

2 cups vegetable stock

3 bay leaves

1 star anise

Bring a large saucepan of water to boil. Place the whole cabbage head inside and cook for 6–8 minutes. Remove and rinse under cold water, reserve the boiling water. Carefully peel 12 outer, larger cabbage leaves away from the head and cut off at the core. Leaves that aren't well cooked can be immersed back in the boiling water for a minute or two to soften them further. Place the leaves on a tray and refrigerate the remaining cabbage for later use.

Preheat oven to 180°C (355°F).

Using your hands, mix the filling ingredients in a bowl until well incorporated.

To make the rolls, take each precooked cabbage leaf and cut away the firmer vein from the bottom for easier rolling. Place 2–3 tbsp of meat mixture in the middle, fold in the sides and roll up tightly. Place seam side down in a deep casserole dish or a baking tray.

Combine diced tomatoes, tomato purée, vegetable stock, bay leaves and star anise in a saucepan and bring to boil. Pour over the cabbage rolls, making sure some of the liquid gets under the rolls. Cover with aluminum foil or an ovenproof lid and cook covered for 20 minutes, and then for an additional 10 minutes uncovered.

Nuts and eggs can be omitted from this recipe. These are traditionally served with some of the tomato broth and a dollop of sour cream.

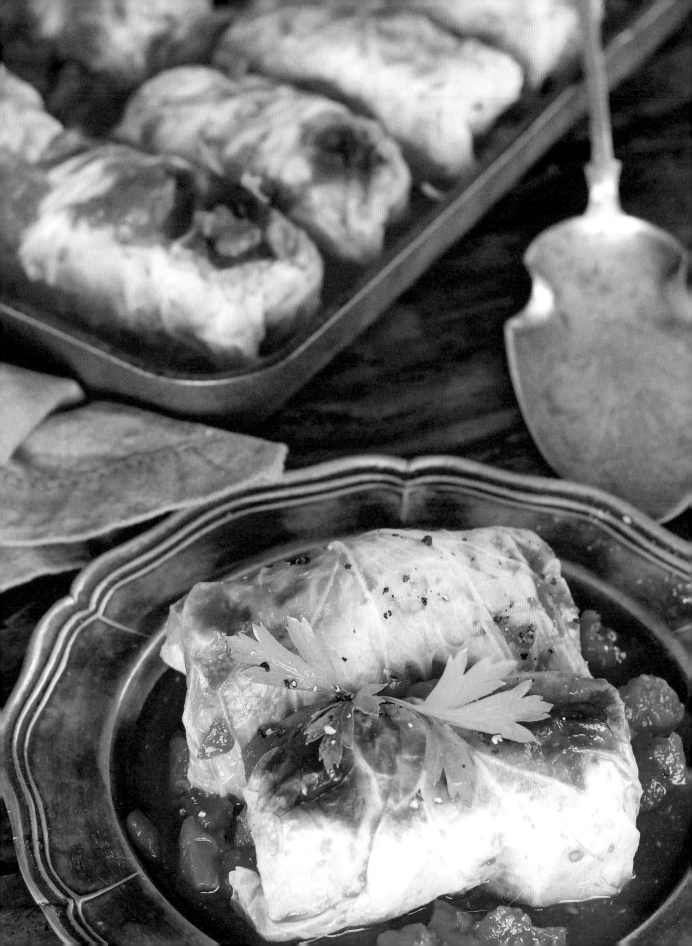

beef skewers

Red meat such as lamb or, even, kangaroo and bison can be used instead of beef.
Serve with roasted sweet potatoes or a nice green salad.

SERVES 6

For the marinade

125ml virgin olive oil

2 tbsp balsamic vinegar

60ml red wine

2 tbsp gluten-free Worcestershire sauce

1 tsp sweet paprika

1/2 tsp smoked paprika

2/3 tsp garlic powder

1/2 tsp coriander seed powder

1 tsp sea salt

1/2 tsp pepper

For the skewers

500g beef fillet, cut into 2–3cm cubes

2 medium courgettes, sliced into 1cm disks

1 small red pepper, cut into 2–3cm squares

1 small yellow pepper, cut into 2–3cm squares

1 red onion, cut into 2–3cm squares

2 tbsp virgin olive oil or spray

8–10 long bamboo skewers, soaked in water for 10 minutes

Mix together the marinade ingredients and coat the beef pieces. Stand aside for 30 minutes to an hour.

Add diced vegetables to the meat and stir through. Thread meat and vegetables onto bamboo skewers, leaving 1cm on each side. Reserve leftover vegetables to grill once the skewers are done.

Preheat a barbecue grill or a large frying pan to high and spray with virgin olive oil or brush with coconut oil. Grill skewers for 3–4 minutes on each side, covering the barbecue hood for 1–2 minutes during that time. Rest skewers for a few minutes before serving.

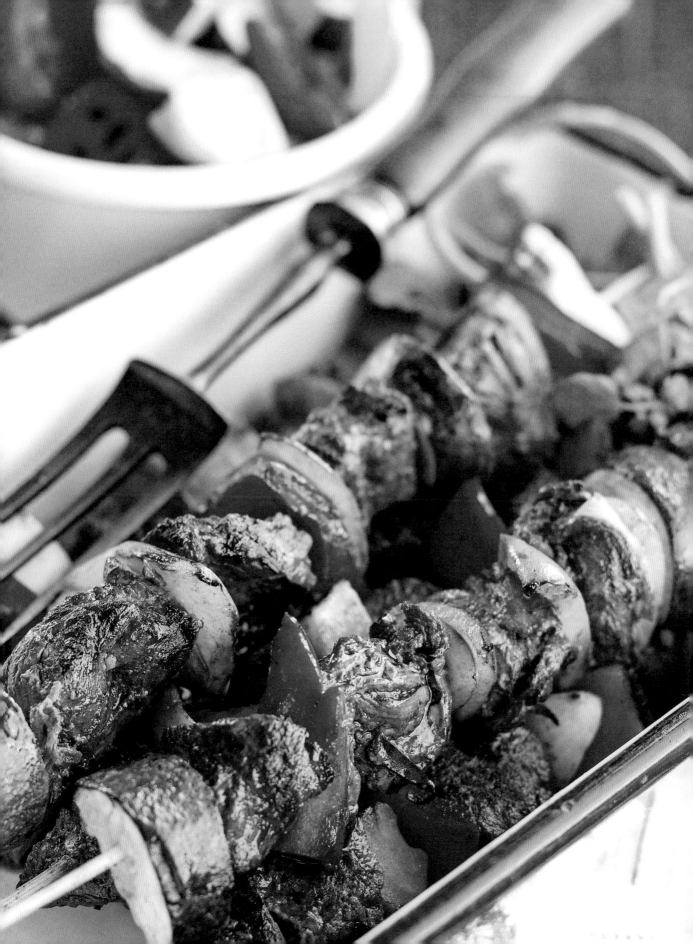

poached coconut chicken salad

You can use this recipe for an easy, no-fuss vegetable side dish with dinner or as a snack or party finger food. It's spicy, yummy and too easy to eat.

SERVES 4

500ml vegetable stock

500ml coconut milk

1 stalk of lemongrass, cut into three

4 kaffir lime leaves

Zest of 1 lime

1 small red chilli, deseeded and sliced

2 tbsp fish sauce

Pinch of sea salt

4 chicken breasts, cut in half

Handful of Thai basil leaves

For coconut dressing

60ml coconut cream

Juice of 1 lime

2 kaffir limes, finely chopped

2 tbsp fish sauce

1 tsp raw honey

For salad

10g mixed lettuce leaves

12.5g fresh coriander (cilantro)

12.5g fresh mint leaves

12.5g Thai basil leaves

1 long red chilli, sliced thinly

1 medium cucumber, sliced thinly

4 spring onions, sliced lengthways

1 mango, peeled and sliced

Preheat oven to 100°C (215°F).

Combine vegetable stock, coconut milk, lemongrass, kaffir lime leaves, lime zest, chilli, fish sauce and salt in a medium saucepan and bring to boil. Place chicken breasts in a casserole dish or deep baking dish and pour the broth over, making sure the meat is covered completely. Place in the oven and cook for 15 to 20 minutes, or until cooked.

Remove chicken to a chopping board to cool and reserve the poaching liquid to make a soup with the next day.

Whisk together the dressing ingredients and set aside. Combine salad ingredients and serve with sliced poached chicken and a couple of tablespoons of coconut dressing, topped with basil leaves.

Remove chilli if avoiding nightshades. You can use any combination of Thai-friendly herbs in this salad – Thai or regular basil, Vietnamese or regular mint, coriander or chives. Visit your local Asian grocer for supplies. Kaffir lime leaves can be replaced with fresh lime peel or some lemongrass.

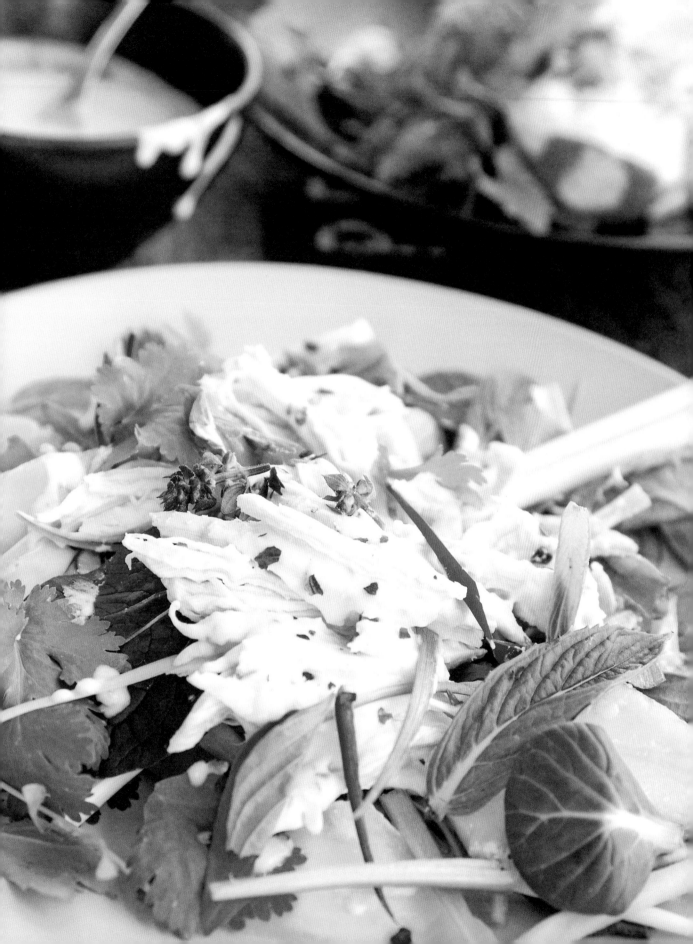

macadamia and herb-crusted pork chops

SERVES 4

6 pork loin chops

Pinch of sea salt and ground black pepper for seasoning

130g macadamia nuts

1 large garlic clove, diced

30g chopped fresh parsley

4 tbsp virgin olive oil

2/3 tsp sea salt

1 tsp ghee

Season pork chops with salt and pepper and leave out of the fridge to come to room temperature. Preheat oven to 180°C (355°F).

Combine macadamia nuts, garlic, parsley, olive oil and salt in a food processor and grind into thick paste.

Heat ghee in a frying pan to sizzling hot and sear the pork chops for 1 minute on each side. Remove to a plate and once slightly cooled down, cover one side with a thin layer of the macadamia crust paste, pressing down with your fingers. Place in a baking tray, crust side up and bake on the middle shelf for 12–15 minutes, until the crust is golden brown and crispy.

harissa almond meatballs

SERVES 3-4

90g blanched almonds

600g lamb mince

2–3 tbsp harissa

110g dried currants or cranberries

1 1/2 tsp sea salt

1/2 tsp ground black pepper

1 tbsp coconut oil

Preheat oven to 175°C (350°F). Place almonds in a medium frying pan and cook over medium heat for 4–5 minutes, stirring frequently, until lightly browned and toasted.

Place almonds in a food processor or use a mortar and pestle to crush them into small crumbs. Combine almond crumbs with ground lamb, harissa, currants, salt and pepper in a mixing bowl. Using wet hands, roll the mixture into small golf ball–sized meatballs and set aside on a plate.

Heat oil in large skillet/frying pan over medium–high heat. In batches, brown the meatballs on all sides. Transfer meatballs to a baking tray and cook in the oven for a further 10–15 minutes. Their internal temperature should be 65–70°C (155–160°F) when they're ready. Serve with tomato or onion relish and lots of vegetables on the side.

A combination of pork and beef mince can be used instead of lamb. You can use a store-bought harissa or make your own. If using dried cranberries or other dried fruit, which are larger than currants, chop them roughly.

chicken larb salad

SERVES 4

For chicken mince

3 tbsp coconut oil

1 stem lemongrass, finely diced

1 long red chilli, finely diced

2 tbsp finely diced fresh coriander stems

3–4 kaffir lime leaves (optional)

Thumb-sized piece of ginger, diced

500g chicken mince

2 garlic cloves, finely diced

1 tsp grated lime zest

3 tbsp fish sauce

1 tbsp coconut aminos

Juice of 1/2 lime

Pinch of sea salt

For the salad

30g raw cashews

Coconut flakes

1/4 large red cabbage, shredded

1 large carrot, grated

1/2 Spanish onion, thinly sliced

2 tbsp fresh coriander leaves

Handful of fresh herbs

1 chopped, fried shallot

For the dressing

2 tbsp extra-virgin olive oil

1 tsp grated palm sugar or honey

3 tbsp lime juice

1 1/2 tbsp fish sauce

1 small red chilli, finely diced

1 tsp sesame oil

Heat coconut oil in a large frying pan or a wok to sizzling hot. Add lemongrass, chilli, coriander stems, kaffir lime leaves and ginger, and stir-fry for a minute until fragrant.

Add chicken mince, garlic and lime zest. Stir and break apart the mince with a wooden spatula until separated into small chunks. Cook for 2–3 minutes until chicken mince has changed colour to white. Add fish sauce, coconut aminos, lime juice and sea salt. Stir through and cook for a further 5 minutes.

Meanwhile, toast cashew nuts for 2–3 minutes in another frying pan. Remove and use a mortar and pestle to grind into smaller crumbs. Add coconut flakes to the same frying pan and cook for a minute, stirring constantly, until toasted and golden brown. Set aside.

Combine the remaining salad ingredients in a mixing bowl. Whisk together the dressing. Add cooked chicken to the salad and mix together with the dressing. Top with toasted cashew nuts, toasted coconut flakes and fried shallot.

Coconut aminos can be purchased in health food shops or ordered online. Use gluten-free Tamari sauce instead or leave out. Fried shallots can be purchased form the Asian section of supermarkets. I try to use coriander stalks when frying chicken as it's a nice way to use up that part of the herb. The best herbs for the salad are fresh coriander, mint, and Thai basil. Visit Eat Drink Paleo website for pictures.

———pulled pork tacos feast———

This was the last main dish I cooked for the cookbook so I invited a few friends over to enjoy my Mexican feast in celebration. We polished off every single bite and the spread got a massive tick of approval! The trick is to plan ahead as the pork takes a few hours to cook. I make the sides in the last hour of pork cooking but you could easily prepare this spread over two days.

SERVES 6–8

For pulled pork

1 tbsp ghee

1kg pork shoulder, cut into 2cm cubes

1 large brown onion, sliced

125ml white wine

500ml chicken stock

1 tsp ground black pepper

1 1/2 tsp smoked paprika

1 1/2 tsp cumin powder

1 tsp coriander seed powder

1 tsp sea salt

3 tbsp tomato purée

3 bay leaves

1 star anise

2 tbsp balsamic vinegar

Zest and juice of 1 lime

1 tbsp coconut sugar or raw honey

20 small cos lettuce leaves, washed and dried

Heat ghee in a large casserole dish until sizzling hot. Add the pork and cook for 4–5 minutes, stirring a couple of times to sear all sides. Add onion, stir through and cook for a minute before adding white wine and the rest of ingredients, except for balsamic vinegar, lime zest and juice, and sweetener. Stir and bring to boil before turning the heat down to low and simmering, covered, for 3 hours. Stir through every half an hour.

At the 2 hours 45 minutes mark, preheat oven to 200°C (390°F). After 3 hours of cooking, mash the pork still in the casserole dish with a potato masher until separated or pull apart with a fork. Add balsamic vinegar, lime zest and coconut sugar or honey and mix through. Transfer to a roasting tray and cook in the oven uncovered for 20–25 minutes, until browned and caramelised. Drizzle with the juice from one lime.

Continued on page 102.

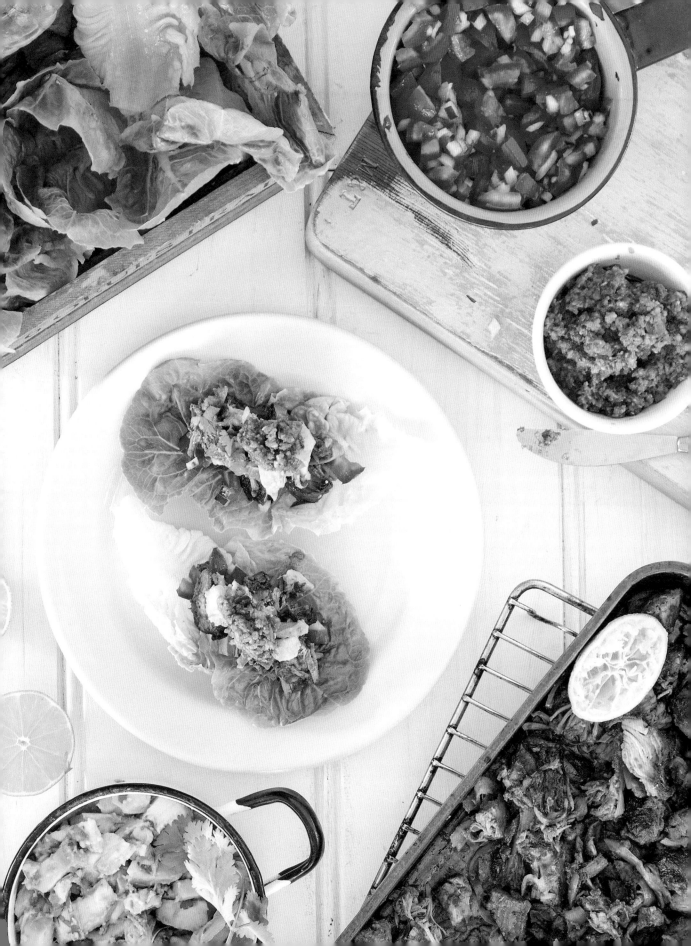

pulled pork tacos feast

For Mexican satay

135g cashews, soaked for 6 hours

2 garlic cloves

3 French shallots, diced

1 long red chilli, chopped (medium heat)

125ml virgin olive oil

2 tsp ground coriander seeds

1 tsp ground coriander

1 tsp smoked paprika

1 tsp sea salt

1 tbsp tomato purée

250ml water

Juice of 1/2 lime

For guacamole

2 ripe avocados

1 tbsp fresh coriander, diced

1/2 garlic clove, crushed

Juice of 1/2 lime

1/2 tsp sea salt

1/2 tsp ground black pepper

For tomato salsa

4 medium tomatoes, quartered and seeds scooped out

1/2 red onion, finely chopped

1 long red chilli, finely diced

2 tbsp red wine vinegar

2 tbsp extra-virgin olive oil

Continued from page 100.

You can prepare this Mexican-flavoured satay sauce the day before or while the pork is cooking. Make sure to soak the cashew nuts for at least 2 hours before using, 6 hours ideally.

Rinse cashew nuts and place in food processor with garlic, shallots and chilli. Grind into small crumbs and transfer to a hot saucepan with virgin olive oil. Add the rest of ingredients, except for water and lime juice. Cook for 3–4 minutes, stirring frequently. Then gradually add the water while stirring the mixture on medium heat. Cook for about 6–8 minutes on low heat until thickened and caramelised. Turn off the heat and stir in the lime juice. Set aside in a serving bowl.

Mash guacamole ingredients together with a fork and serve in a bowl.

Dice tomatoes into small cubes and combine with the rest of the salsa ingredients in a bowl.

Serve pulled pork in cos lettuce leaves, topped with guacamole, tomato salad and a small dollop of spicy Mexican satay sauce.

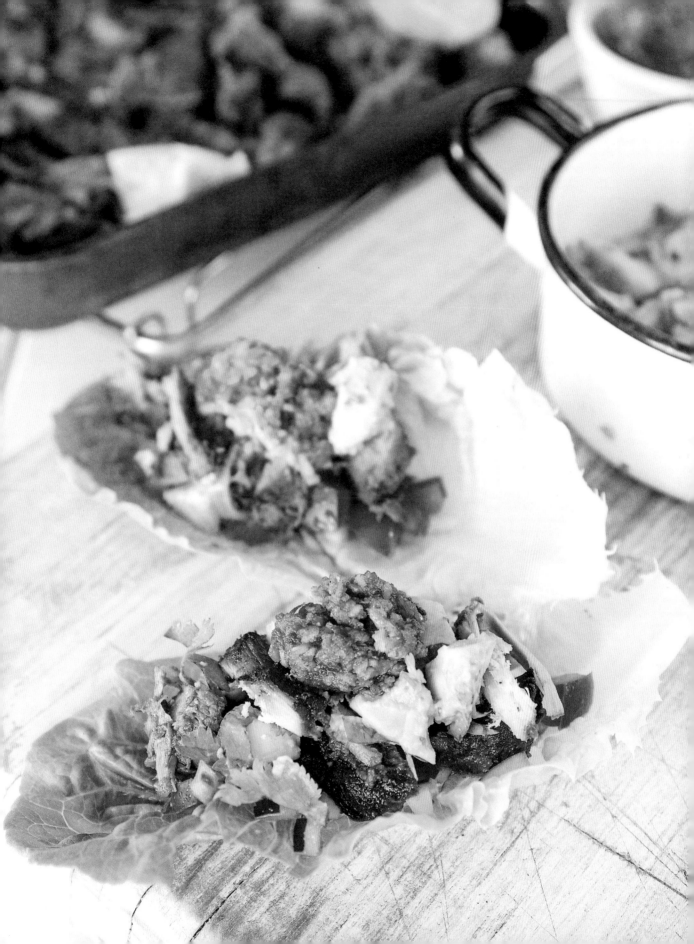

asian chicken cakes

Fragrant and full of oriental, zesty flavours, these chicken cakes are like savoury candy. Make as part of an Asian-inspired dinner party or as a main dish with sautéed greens and cucumber salad. Dip in my Asian Twang dressing from page 192 before popping in your mouth.

MAKES 12–14 CAKES

800g chicken mince

2 eggs

1 long red chilli, finely chopped

2 garlic cloves, finely chopped

2 tbsp fresh coriander, chopped

1 tbsp Thai basil leaves, chopped

3 tbsp green onion, chopped

Thumb-sized piece of fresh ginger, grated

2 tbsp fish sauce

1 tsp sesame oil

Zest of 1 lime

2 tbsp lime juice

2 tbsp coconut oil for cooking

To serve

2 medium cucumbers, sliced into ribbons

Handful of Thai basil

Combine all ingredients in a mixing bowl and use your hand to mash and incorporate. Roll into golf ball-sized rounds and flatten slightly.

Heat coconut oil to sizzling hot and cook chicken cakes on medium heat for 5–7 minutes on each side. Serve with fresh cucumber, Thai basil and a spicy dipping sauce on the side.

You can use the same recipe for pork and beef mince instead of chicken. Cooked cakes will last for 2–3 days in the fridge and for up to a month in the freezer. They can be added to curry sauces and broken into chunks for Asian omelettes.

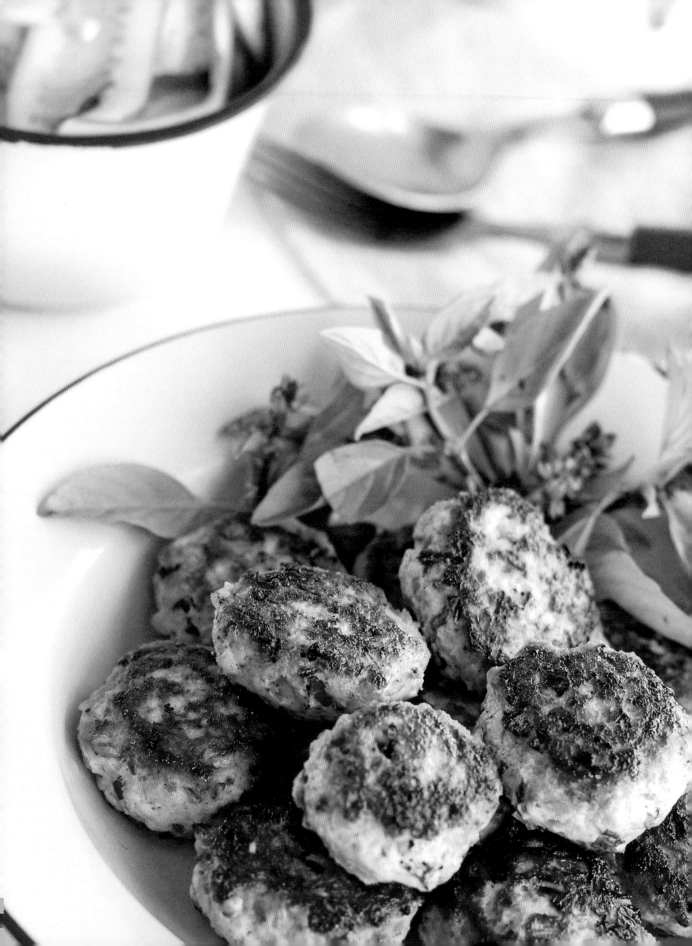

mustard thyme quail

My favourite thing about quail is that you can have the whole bird to yourself and pull it apart, biting the succulent, tasty meat right off the bones. Nothing like licking oozing juices off your fingers.

SERVES 5

For the marinade

1/2 tsp turmeric

1 tsp Dijon mustard

2 tbsp fresh thyme leaves

2 garlic cloves, diced

1/2 tsp ground black pepper

1 1/2 tsp sea salt

Zest of 1 lemon

2 tbsp lemon juice

125ml virgin olive oil

For the quail

5 whole quails

10 sprigs of fresh thyme

5 garlic cloves, peeled

5 slices of lemon

5 pieces of 30cm long butcher's string

Preheat oven 190°C (375°F).

Place all marinade ingredients in a food processor and process until well incorporated. Smother all over the quail bodies and inside the cavities. Stand aside for 15 minutes.

Stuff 2 sprigs of thyme, a garlic clove and a slice of lemon inside each quail. Tie the legs with butcher's string and place in a deep roasting tray. Cook in the oven for 35 minutes. Remove and leave to rest under aluminum foil for 5–10 minutes before serving.

You can use the same marinade to roast chicken, spatchcock or pigeon birds. Bake leeks and carrots on the lower shelf for a perfect side dish.

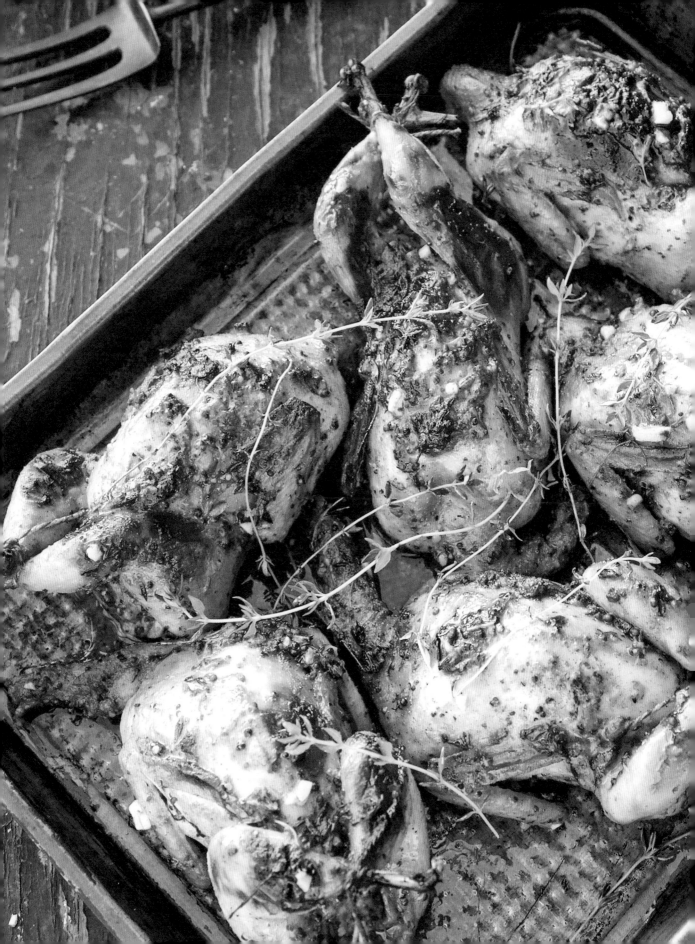

lemon harissa lamb cutlets

Serve these lamb cutlets with roasted pumpkin and a rocket salad. Omit pine nuts if allergic. Ask your butcher to French trim the lamb rack. You can prepare harissa ahead of time.

SERVES 2–3

1/2 tsp cumin powder

1/2 tsp sweet paprika

1 tsp sea salt

2/3 tsp ground black pepper

1 rack of lamb cutlets, French trimmed

1 tsp coconut oil

2 tbsp pine nuts

60ml lemon harissa (page 176)

2 tbsp fresh coriander leaves

1 long red chilli, thinly sliced

Preheat oven to 180°C (355°F).

Mix together the cumin, paprika, salt and pepper, and rub over the lamb rack. Heat coconut oil in a frying pan and sear the lamb on each side for 3 minutes, until browned.

Place in a roasting tray and cook in the oven for 12 minutes. At the same time, place pine nuts on another baking tray and toast in the oven for 2 minutes. Remove lamb from the oven and rest for 5 minutes before slicing in between the bones, into individual cutlets.

While the cutlets are in the oven, prepare the harissa from page 176. Serve cutlets on a chopping board drizzled with lemon harissa and sprinkled with pine nuts, fresh coriander and sliced chilli.

curried lamb cutlets

SERVES 3

1 1/2 tbsp curry powder

1/2 tsp ground coriander

1/2 tsp ground cumin

1/2 tsp chilli powder or flakes

2 garlic cloves, finely chopped

1 tbsp coconut aminos

125ml coconut cream

2/3 tsp sea salt

12 French-trimmed lamb cutlets

1 tbsp coconut oil

Combine all ingredients except the lamb and coconut oil in a bowl. Coat the cutlets in the mixture and marinate for 15–20 minutes.

Heat coconut oil in a large frying pan over medium–high heat. In batches, cook lamb cutlets for 3 minutes on each side for medium to medium-rare. Rest for a few minutes before serving.

Any leftover marinade can be cooked for a minute and used on top of the cutlets.

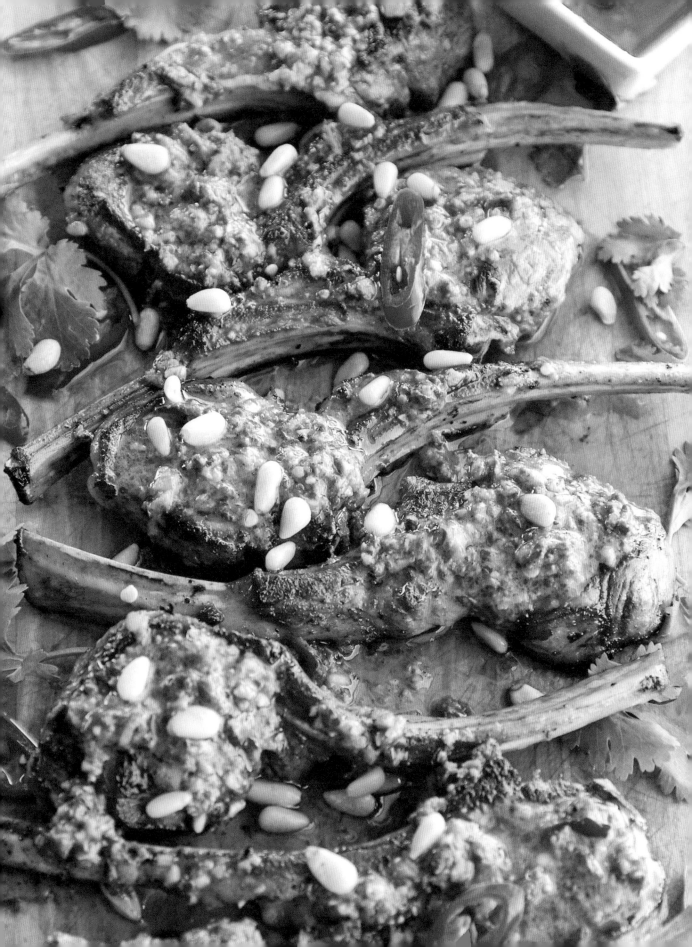

my famous lasagne

This is the most popular recipe on the Eat Drink Paleo website, so I simply had to include it in my cookbook. It's delicious! No other commentary needed.

SERVES 6

For beef and tomato sauce

2 tbsp virgin olive oil

1 brown onion, diced

1 tsp sea salt, plus a pinch extra

1 tsp ghee

500g grass-fed beef mince

185ml dry red wine

3 garlic cloves, finely chopped

2/3 tsp black pepper

2/3 tsp sweet paprika

750ml tomato passata

For lasagne layers

1 large aubergine, sliced into 1cm thick discs

1 tsp sea salt

2 tbsp virgin olive oil

2 parsnips, peeled and sliced thinly

5 tbsp virgin olive oil

2 tsp ghee

10g torn fresh basil leaves

5–6 button mushrooms, sliced

50g baby spinach leaves

3 medium courgettes, sliced vertically into thin ribbons

390g ricotta cheese (optional)

2–3 tbsp grated Parmesan cheese

Cherry tomatoes and basil leaves to garnish

For the sauce, heat 2 tbsp of olive oil and sauté onion with a pinch of salt for 5 minutes. Add 1 tsp of ghee and the beef and bring the heat up to high. Use a spatula or a potato masher to stir and break the mince apart into small pieces, as it tends to clump together during cooking. Cook for about 5–6 minutes, until browned.

Add red wine, garlic, pepper, paprika and salt and fry for 3–4 minutes. Add tomato passata, bring to boil and turn the heat down to simmering temperature. Cook for 10 minutes. Meanwhile, sprinkle aubergine with salt and set aside for 10 minutes to draw out juices. Rinse and pat dry. Heat oven to 180°C (355°F).

Brush the bottom of an oven dish with olive oil. Place a layer of parsnips on the bottom, overlapping each other. Bake in the oven for 10 minutes.

In another frying pan, heat 2 tbsp olive oil and 1 tsp ghee. Fry the aubergine in batches for 3 minutes on each side, until browned. Add more olive oil and ghee as you go along.

Remove baking tray from the oven and layer the lasagne in the following order: pre-cooked parsnips, 1/3 of tomato meat sauce, aubergine slices, fresh basil leaves, mushrooms, the rest of the sauce, baby spinach, courgette, drizzle of olive oil and some cracked black pepper. Press down evenly and cook in the oven, at 180°C (355°F), for 35–40 minutes. If using ricotta and grated Parmesan cheese, add on top of the lasagne at the 20 minutes cooking-time mark. Increase the heat to 200°C (390°F) for the last 10–15 minutes. Garnish with fresh basil and a few cherry tomatoes. Serve with a mixed salad.

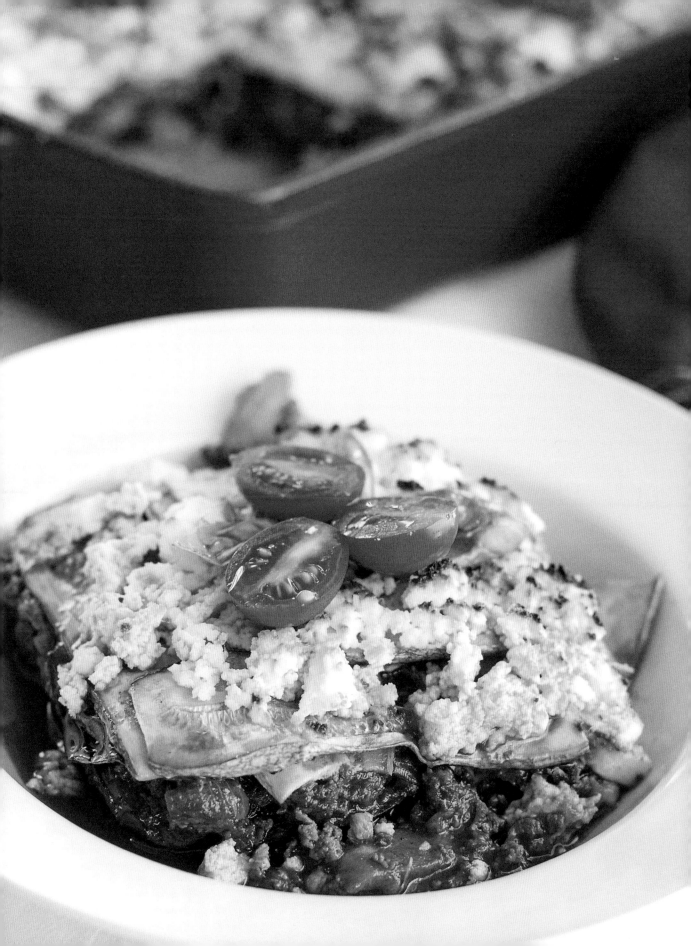

filet mignon, leeks and mushrooms

Filet mignon, also known as tenderloin steak, is one of the most tender cuts of beef and requires little effort in the kitchen. Many believe that it's sacrilege to cook it beyond medium or medium-rare, and that it needs no marinating. All it needs is a couple of beautiful complementary sides.

SERVES 4

For leeks

2 tbsp coconut oil

2 leeks, sliced

2/3 tsp seeded mustard

Pinch of sea salt

For mushrooms

40g dry porcini mushrooms

2 tbsp virgin olive oil

1 tsp ghee + 1/2 tsp at the end

225–300g sliced button mushrooms

3 cloves garlic, diced

2/3 tsp sea salt

1 tsp grated lemon zest

125ml white wine

125ml porcini water (reserved after soaking porcini mushrooms)

1 tsp tapioca flour/starch

1 tbsp lemon juice

For filet mignon steaks

2 beef filet mignon steaks (150g each)

1/2 tsp sea salt

1/2 tsp ground black pepper

1 tsp coconut oil

Soak dry porcini mushrooms in boiling hot water for 10 minutes. Remove mushrooms and reserve the liquid.

Take the steaks out of the fridge, sprinkle with a little salt and pepper and set aside to come to room temperature.

For the leeks, heat the coconut oil in a medium saucepan or a frying pan to medium hot and cook leeks together with mustard and a pinch of salt for 12–15 minutes, stirring occasionally.

Meanwhile, heat olive oil and 1 tsp of ghee in another frying pan. Add porcini and fresh mushrooms, garlic, salt and lemon zest and cook for 3–4 minutes until slightly browned. Add white wine and porcini mushroom water and turn the heat to high to bring to boil. Then simmer for 3–4 minutes before adding 1 tsp of tapioca flour dissolved in a little warm water, lemon juice and another 1/2 tsp of ghee. Stir through to thicken the sauce and turn off the heat. Transfer to a bowl.

Heat coconut oil to in a frying pan to sizzling hot. Cook steaks for 3–4 minutes on each side for medium to medium-rare. Rest for 2 minutes before serving. Top each steak with a large spoonful of coconut leeks and sautéed mushrooms to serve.

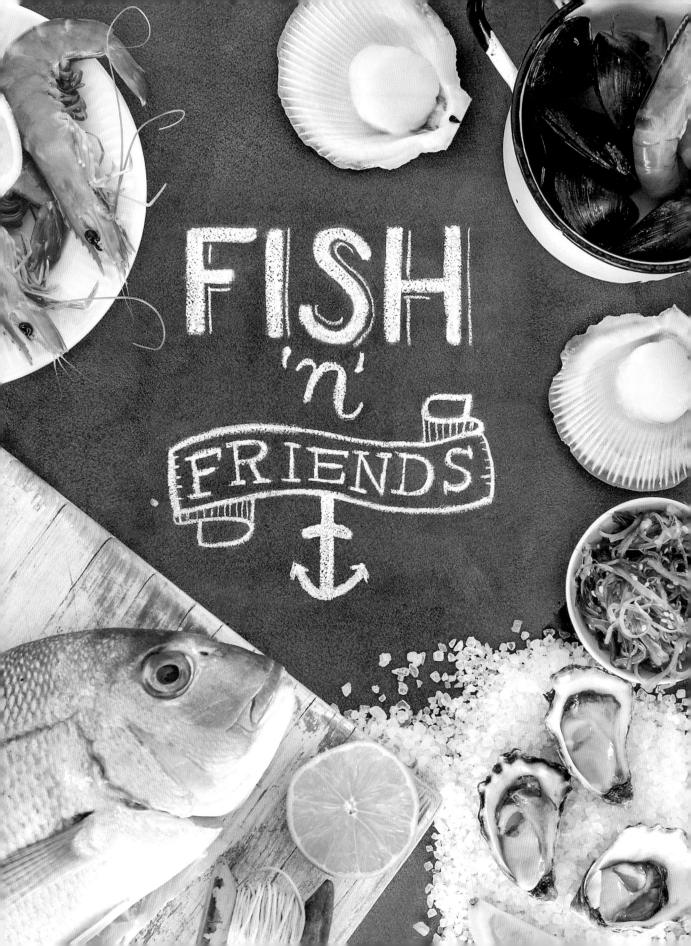

mackerel plaki

Take a trip to a Greek island with this traditional baked fish recipe. The Greeks often make it with mackerel but any other medium-sized whole fish can be used. Mackerel has a pretty strong taste but it's beautifully mellowed, and at the same time complemented by sweet tomatoes and peppers, garlic, onions and wine. This recipe uses larger mackerel fish but you can easily make this with six to eight smaller fish.

SERVES 2

2 small brown onions, peeled and sliced

1 medium red pepper and 1 meduim yellow pepper

4 tbsp extra-virgin olive oil

2 mackerel, cleaned and gutted

3 garlic cloves, finely chopped

2 tbsp parsley

1 punnet/tray cherry tomatoes, cut in half

3 fresh bay leaves

2 medium carrots, peeled and thinly sliced

Juice and zest of 1 lemon

1 tsp sea salt or Celtic salt

1/2 tsp black pepper

250ml dry white wine

You can add olives, sliced fennel and other herbs such as oregano or basil

Season onions and peppers with a pinch of salt. Heat the olive oil in a pan and cook the onions and peppers on low to medium heat for around 15 minutes until softened and slightly caramelised.

Preheat the oven to 180°C (355°F). Line a deep baking tray with two pieces of aluminum foil, making sure the sides are well covered.

Stuff the fish with some of the garlic and parsley. Place half the cooked onion and red peppers on the bottom of the tray and top with half the cherry tomatoes, a little more garlic, bay leaves, and half of each of the carrots, lemon zest and lemon juice. Sprinkle with pepper and salt. Place mackerel on top and cover with the rest of ingredients. Drizzle with the remaining lemon juice and pour over the wine. Cover with a piece of foil and bake for 20 minutes, letting the fish steam inside. Remove the top layer of foil and bake for a further 20 minutes uncovered to allow it to caramelise and brown.

Tip: Keep the oven steady at 180°C (355°F) and use the middle shelf.

Serve with a large green salad or barbecued vegetables such as courgette, asparagus and sweet potato.

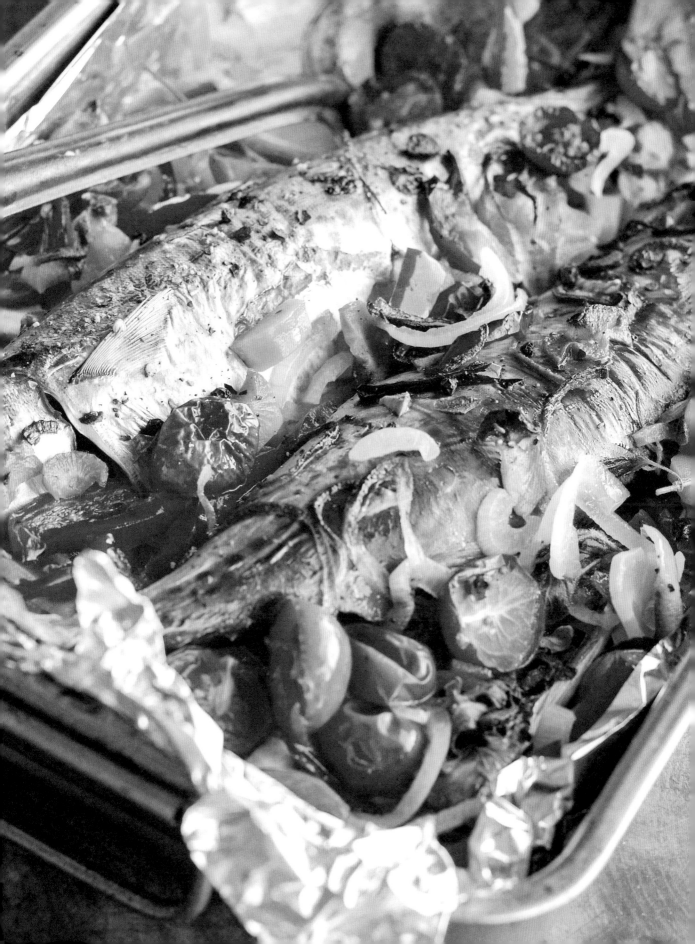

basque sardines

This dish is inspired by the grilled sardines I had in Biarritz, a beautiful coastal town in the Basque region of France. The original dish didn't have the same seasoning as this one and the sardines were grilled whole but I feel it still captures that gorgeous warm evening at the fisherman's wharf with my best friend, combining the taste of the sea with Basque flavours of paprika, garlic, olive oil and garlic.

SERVES 2

10 sardines, cleaned and gutted

2 garlic cloves, finely chopped

3 tbsp olive or macadamia oil

2 tbsp chopped fresh parsley

1 tsp sweet paprika

2/3 tsp sea salt

Pinch of black pepper

Ghee for cooking

Lemon juice

To flatten the sardines and remove the backbone, open out the gut cavity and lay the fish on the chopping board skin side up. Press down on the backbone with the palm of your hand from the head to the tail. Turn the fish over and peel off the backbone. You can use a pair of scissors to cut it out and remove the head. Don't worry if you have a few small bones remaining. Alternatively, ask your fishmonger to do it.

Cook garlic in oil in a small frying pan on low heat for 4–5 minutes until golden brown. Stir a few times to avoid burning. Remove to a paper towel to drain some of the oil, as we don't want too much moisture.

Mix fried garlic with chopped parsley, paprika, salt and pepper and set aside in a bowl.

Heat 1 tbsp of ghee in a grill pan until sizzling hot. Place flattened sardines skin side down and cook for 2–3 minutes. Carefully scrape and flip over using a metal spatula and cook for a further 30 seconds, just to brown the inside slightly.

Serve sardines sprinkled with parsley and paprika seasoning and lemon juice. This dish pairs nicely with a glass of good quality rosé wine.

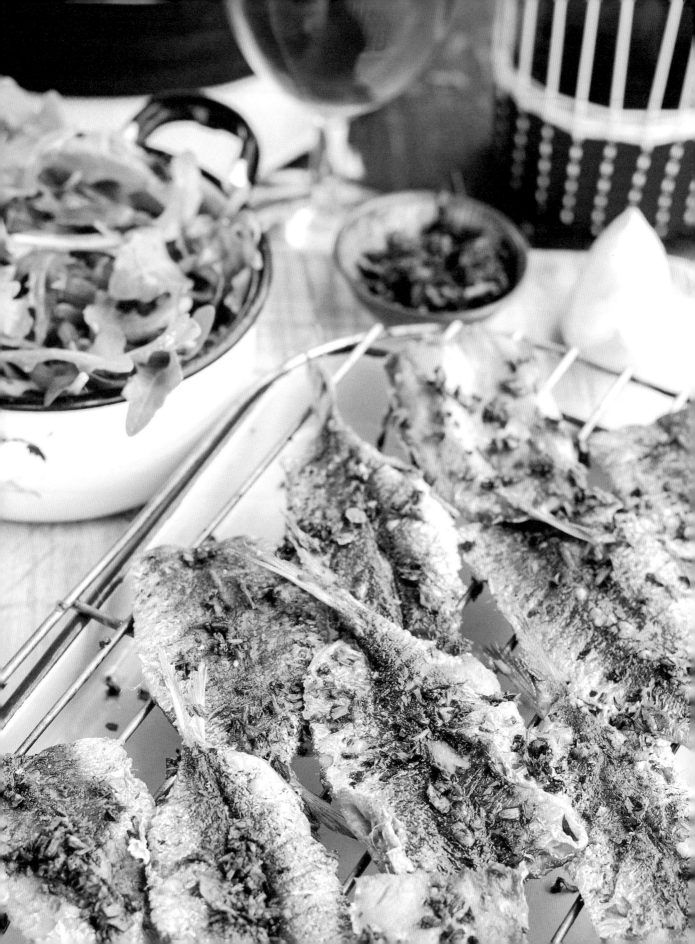

oysters five ways

Succulent, juicy, salty and full of iron, zinc, copper, vitamin D and good omega-3 fatty acids – oysters are on the top of both nutritional and food connoisseurs' must-have lists. Next time you get a platter to go with a crisp glass of white wine, try one of these dressings inspired by my favourite world cuisines. Simply dice and mix all ingredients in a bowl and serve with oysters.

ENOUGH FOR A DOZEN OYSTERS

MEXICAN

4 jalapeno slices from the jar, chopped

1 tbsp chopped fresh coriander

1/4 tsp cumin powder

1 1/2 tbsp lime juice

2 tbsp extra-virgin olive oil

FRENCH

1 small French shallot, finely diced

1 tbsp red wine vinegar

1/4 tsp ground coriander seed

1 1/2 tbsp extra-virgin olive oil

Pinch of salt

ASIAN

1 tsp grated or finely diced fresh ginger

1 tsp finely diced long red chilli

1 tsp sesame oil

1 tbsp lime juice

1/2 tsp grated palm sugar/honey

1 tsp fish sauce

1 1/2 tbsp extra-virgin olive oil

ITALIAN

1/2 medium tomato, diced and seeds removed

2 green or Kalamata olives, chopped

1/2 tbsp chopped fresh parsley or basil

1 tbsp balsamic or white wine vinegar

2 tbsp extra-virgin olive oil

Pinch of salt

RUSSIAN

1 tbsp diced cucumber

1 tsp chopped fresh dill

1 tbsp lemon juice

1 1/2 tbsp extra-virgin olive oil

Pinch of salt and pepper

Fish roe on top

MEXICAN

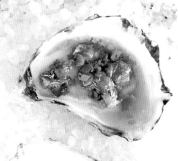

ASIAN

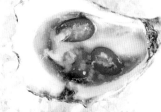

RUSSKI

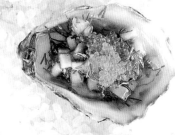

FRENCH

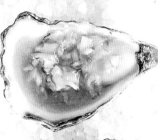

Italian

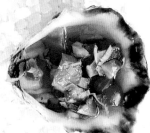

lemongrass & white wine mussels

This dish is somewhat special as it's one of the first meals my partner ever cooked for me and it earned him quite a few brownie points. He still cooks it for me today and I love it so much I asked if I could adapt and use the recipe in the cookbook. It's so fresh and full of flavour; plus, mussels are very nutritious.

SERVES 2

1 tbsp coconut oil or butter

3 spring onions, chopped

1/2 long red chilli, sliced

1 stalk lemongrass, finely diced, pale part only

2 garlic cloves, chopped

375ml dry white wine

1 1/2 tbsp fish sauce

250ml vegetable stock

1kg mussels, cleaned

Handful of fresh mint

Handful of Thai or regular basil

Lemon for garnish and final drizzle

> When buying mussels look for closed shells and, if open, check if they close or move when you tap or squeeze them, which indicates that the mussel is alive. Avoid any mussels that smell 'fishy', look open or have broken shells, as they might be dead inside. The colour of the flesh indicates whether the mussel is female (orange meat) or male (white meat).

Heat a large soup pot or a wide pan over medium–low heat and melt the butter. Make sure you have a lid to cover the pan with. Add spring onion, chilli, lemongrass and garlic and sauté for a minute or two until everything softens.

Turn the heat up and add white wine and fish sauce. Let the liquid bubble away for about 30 seconds before adding the vegetable stock. Bring back to boil and add the mussels. Stir to cover all mussels with the broth before covering the pan with a lid and cooking the lot for 5–6 minutes on medium heat. Give it another stir half-way through to rotate the bottom and top layer of the mussels. Turn the heat off when most of the mussels have opened up.

Finally, toss through the herbs, making sure they get all the way to the bottom. Drizzle a couple of tablespoons of lemon juice over the top. Serve in a pot with tongs and a spoon for the broth. Normally, mussels are served with a fresh baguette or some thick-cut fries to soak up the liquid but you can also serve a side of steamed broccoli or snow peas to add to the broth once all the mussels are gone.

Tip: Mussel shells will usually open when cooked. According to the Australian Mussels Industry Association, it's an urban myth that unopened cooked mussels should be discarded (read more on their website). When cooked, the mussels should be plump, juicy and have a fresh taste of the sea.

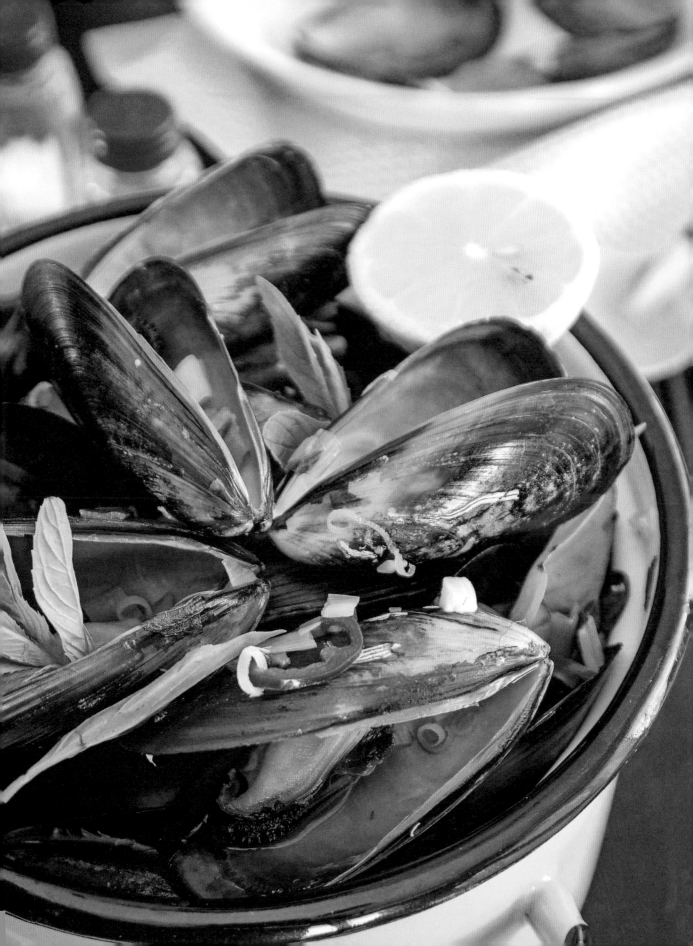

macadamia-crusted fish fingers

This is my modern take on an all-time favourite dish. The fish is partially covered with the crumbed mixture of healthy macadamia nuts, parsley and garlic, making it more delicate and fragrant than regular crumbed fish. Tartare sauce is replaced with creamy red cabbage coleslaw, spiked with the faint aniseed aroma of tarragon, which complements the fish beautifully. It's all a little bit spring and a little bit French, really.

SERVES 2

For the fish fingers

500g white fish fillets such as pollock or coley

3/4 tsp sea salt

130g macadamia nuts

2 garlic cloves, chopped roughly

Zest of 1 lemon

2 tbsp fresh chopped parsley

2 tbsp virgin olive oil

Pinch of black pepper

Lemon wedges to serve

For the coleslaw

1/4 red cabbage, thinly sliced

1 medium carrot, peeled and grated

1/2 medium red onion, thinly sliced

1 tbsp mayonnaise

10–15 fresh tarragon leaves

1 tbsp white wine vinegar

1 tbsp extra-virgin olive oil

Pinch of salt and pepper

Preheat oven to 200°C (390°F). Slice fish fillets into 1–2cm wide strips, sprinkle with a little salt and set aside.

Combine all other ingredients for the fish and process into a fine crumbly mixture using a food processor or blender. Coat each fish slice in a layer of crumb mixture, using your fingers to press mixture onto the fish.

Grease a baking tray with some coconut or virgin olive oil and place a piece of baking paper on top. Place crumbed fish fillets on top, leaving some space in between. Bake for 12 minutes or until the crumbed mixture turns golden brown and crisp.

Meanwhile, combine all coleslaw ingredients in a bowl. Serve with fish fingers.

Learn how to make mayonnaise on page 191.

You can bake whole crumbed fish fillets instead of individual smaller strips. Tarragon can be omitted or replaced with fresh dill, which also goes well with fish and seafood. Those avoiding eggs can leave out the mayonnaise and add a little extra lemon juice and olive oil for the salad dressing.

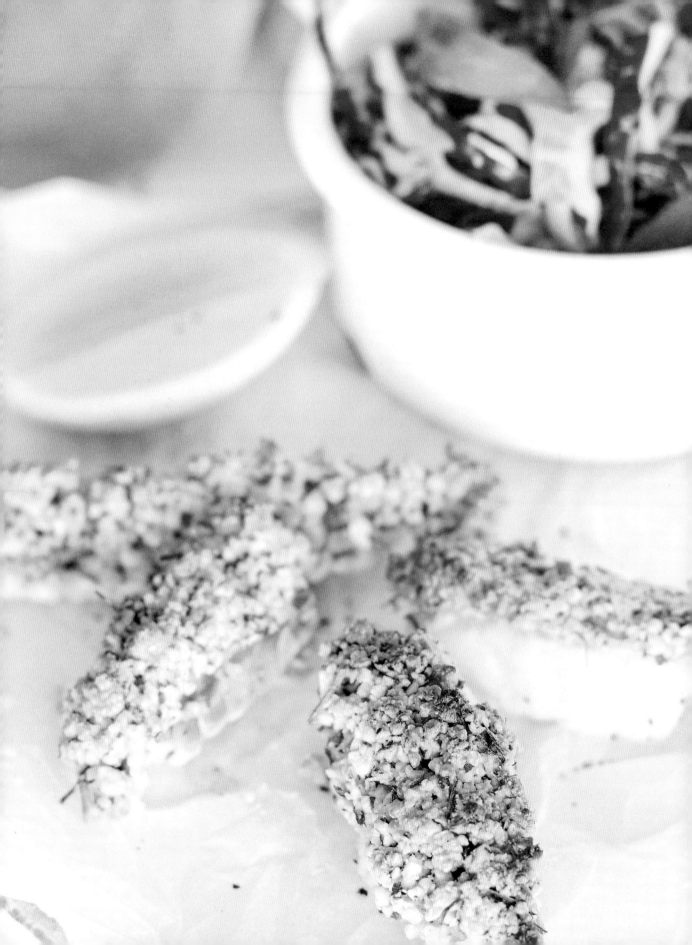

lime & coriander butter scallops

Serve this dish to your guests or as a special starter at a family Sunday lunch and take everyone on a mini trip to the Caribbean. You can't go wrong with the combination of sweet, plump scallops and fresh citrus butter.

MAKES 12 SHELLS

2 tbsp Lime & Coriander Butter (page 194)

12 scallops in shells

1/2 lime, juice only

Pinch of black pepper

Good pinch of sea salt

Pre-heat oven to 200°C (390°F) and then switch to the grill function.

Scoop half a teaspoon of lime and coriander butter on top of each scallop. Place the shells on a flat tray, and cook under a hot grill for 4–5 minutes. Squeeze over some lime juice and sprinkle a little sea salt and pepper over the top and serve hot.

> Those who don't like coriander (some people claim it tastes like soap) can use parsley instead. If avoiding all dairy, use olive oil instead of butter and make a salsa-like dressing instead.

lime & sesame tuna tartare

SERVES 2

1 tsp lime zest

Juice of 1 lime

1 tbsp coconut aminos

1 tbsp fish sauce

1 tsp sesame oil

1 tsp extra-virgin olive oil

Pinch of sea salt and pepper

250g sashimi-grade tuna

1 tbsp finely diced chives

1 tbsp toasted sesame seeds

1 avocado, mashed

1 tbsp lime or lemon juice

1 tbsp chopped coriander

Generous pinch of sea salt

Combine the first 7 ingredients in a bowl and set aside.

Slice tuna into strips and then into small cubes. Add to the bowl with the dressing, chives and sesame seeds. Combine and set aside.

Combine avocado with lime juice, coriander and salt. Divide tuna mixture between small plates or bowls and top with the avocado mash. Serve with sliced radishes and lettuce leaves, which you can use to wrap the tartare.

You can serve these with my sesame and tahini crackers from page 172 or with sweet potato chips.

> Coconut aminos can be replaced with 1 tbsp Tamari sauce and 1/2 tsp honey. Other sashimi grade fish can be used instead of tuna.

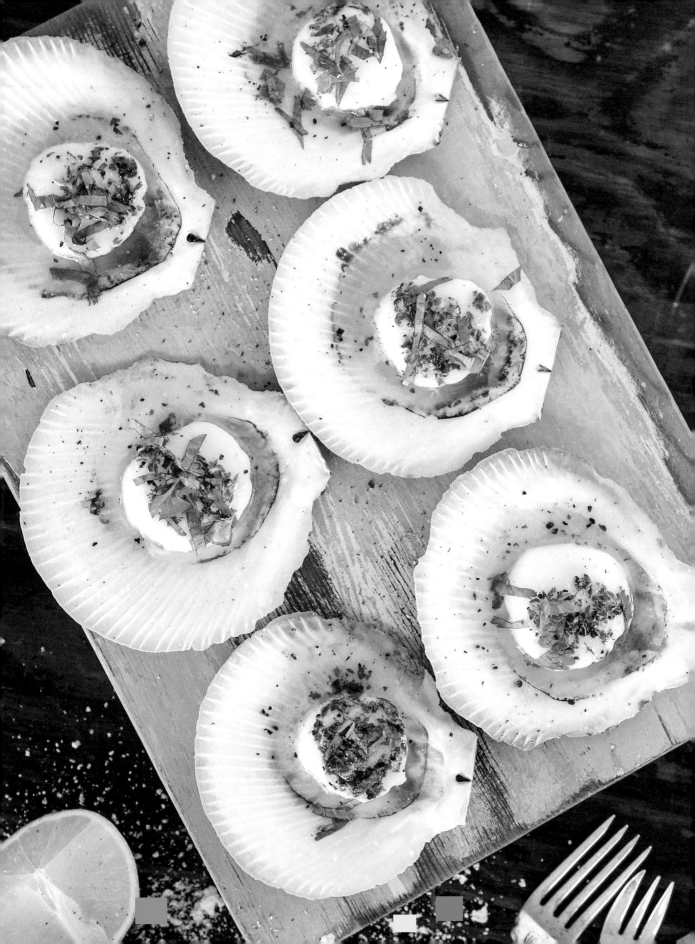

red curry prawns

Leave your manners at the door and get a bowl of water ready because you'll be licking your fingers like it's going out of style with this dish. This is my favourite way to prepare fresh prawns and my friends absolutely love it. I like to marinate and cook the prawns in shells because it gives them a rich flavour when grilled and protects the flesh from overcooking.

SERVES 4

For the red curry paste

2 shallots, diced

3 garlic cloves, roughly chopped

2 long red chillies, chopped

1 stalk lemongrass, sliced

1 tbsp galangal, peeled and grated

1 tbsp fresh turmeric, peeled and grated

6 kaffir lime leaves

2 tbsp chopped coriander stalks

1 tbsp fish sauce

2 tbsp virgin olive oil

1/2 tsp palm or coconut sugar

To marinate prawns

700g fresh king prawns

125ml coconut cream

Pinch of salt

Juice of 1/2 lime

To make the curry paste, place all ingredients in a food processor and purée into as smooth a paste as possible, for about 2–3 minutes. Keep in the fridge, in an airtight container, covered with a layer of olive oil for up to seven days.

To prepare the prawns, grip the body of the prawn in one hand and twist the head off with the other (you can save the heads to make stock). To butterfly a prawn, make a deep cut along the belly of the prawn almost all the way to the shell but not quite. Open it out and press it down so it's flat. The shell will crunch and break a little. Remove the intestinal tract – the dark vein – running down the length of the prawn and rinse the body.

Use your hands to toss the butterflied prawns in 2 tbsp of curry paste, coconut cream, salt and lime juice until well coated. Leave to marinate in the fridge for 4–5 hours.

Pre-heat a barbecue or a grill until sizzling hot and spray or brush with some oil. Place the prawns flesh side down first and cook for 3 minutes. Turn over and cook on the shell side for another minute. If you don't butterfly the prawns, cook for 2–3 minutes on each side. Serve with freshly squeezed lime juice and fresh coriander and sliced chilli.

Like all shellfish, prawns go off quickly, so keep in the fridge wrapped in their original packaging or submerged in water in a sealed container. Eat within 24 hours of purchase. Use the remaining paste to make a curry or soup.

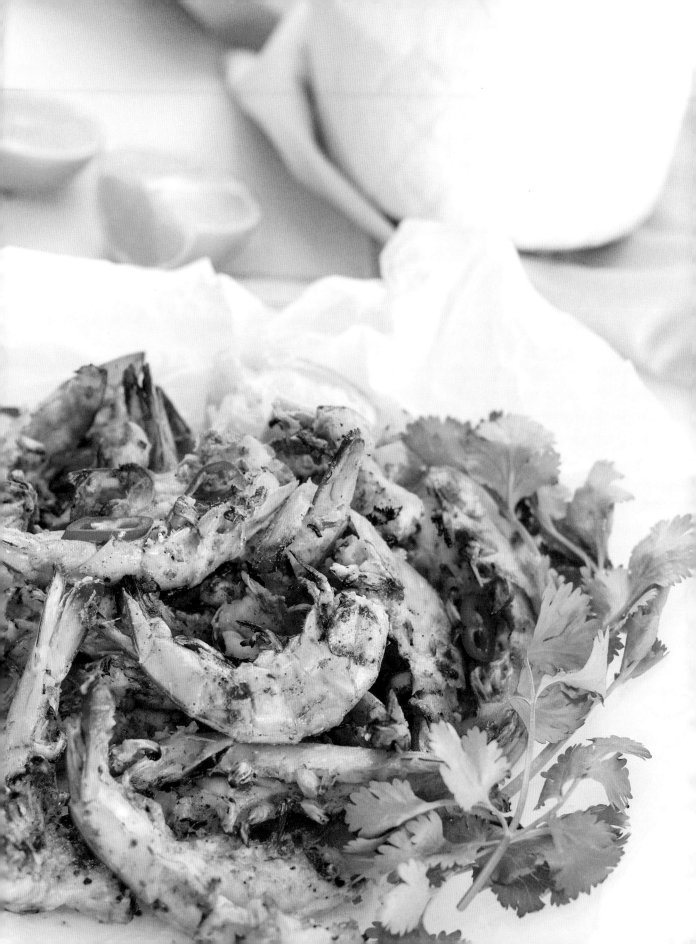

rosemary salt-baked fish

A traditionally Spanish method of baking fish in salt keeps the flesh perfectly cooked and moist, and although it might seem like the dish will turn out extremely salty, the fish absorbs only a subtle flavour of salt and rosemary, leaving the taste of the flesh intact. It looks impressive, almost theatrical, when you carve away chunks of the salt blanket when serving the fish, but the actual cooking method is ridiculously simple.

SERVES 4

1kg table salt

2 tbsp chopped fresh or dry rosemary

60ml water

1 egg (only for the salt blanket)

1 whole red snapper

Couple of rosemary sprigs

Preheat oven to 200°C (390°F). Grease a flat baking tray with virgin olive oil and place a sheet of baking paper over the top.

In a large bowl, mix salt with chopped rosemary, water and egg.

Wash and pat dry the snapper. Place a layer of salt mixture in the middle of the baking tray. Place the fish on top, with a couple of rosemary sprigs inside its cavity, and cover with a layer of salt, about 1cm thick, on all sides. The salt mixture will be slightly moist, so you can mould it around the fish. Bake for 20–25 minutes, until the salt crust has turned golden brown and hard.

Serve inside the salt blanket with lemon wedges on the side. Carve the salt blanket on the table; it will break away in large pieces. Peel the scales away and enjoy the moist, flavoursome fish.

Serve with rocket, fennel, orange and olive salad.

When buying the snapper, ask your fishmonger to remove the guts and clean the fish but to leave the scales on. This is a protective layer from the salt flavour. Once cooked, the fish will stay warm inside the salt blanket for a little while.

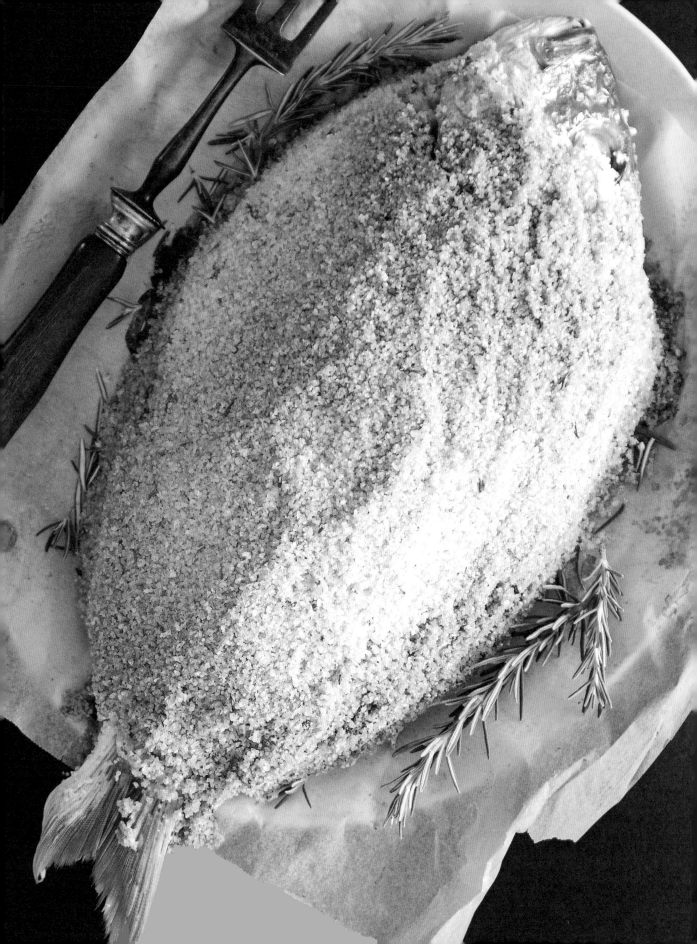

mexican tuna steaks

SERVES 2

For the tuna steaks

2 tuna steaks, 150g each, 1cm thick

Pinch of sea salt and black pepper

Drizzle of olive oil

1 tsp ground coriander seeds

2 tbsp macadamia oil or coconut oil

1 tsp butter (use ghee if avoiding dairy)

Zest and juice of 1 lime (reserve some juice for avocado)

For the sweet peppers

3 tbsp virgin olive oil

1 medium red onion, sliced

1 red pepper, sliced into thin strips

2/3 tsp sweet paprika

2/3 tsp cumin powder

1 large garlic clove, chopped

1 tbsp apple cider vinegar

Pinch of sea salt

Good pinch of red chilli flakes

2 tbsp water

For avocado

1 large, ripe avocado

2 tbsp chopped fresh coriander

Pinch of sea salt

Juice of about 1/2 a lime

Wash and pat dry tuna steaks, sprinkle with a little salt, pepper and drizzle with olive oil. Set aside to bring to room temperature.

For the sweet peppers, heat oil in a frying pan, add sliced onion and red pepper, cover with a lid and cook for 5 minutes, stirring a couple of times. Add paprika, cumin, garlic, apple cider vinegar, a pinch of salt, chilli flakes, and about 2 tablespoons of water. Stir and cook for a further 4–5 minutes until softened and slightly browned. Remove to a plate or use a different frying pan for the tuna steaks.

Grind coriander seeds in a mortar and pestle. Heat oil and butter or ghee to sizzling hot. Add coriander seed powder and lime zest and stir through the oil.

Keeping the heat high, add tuna steaks and then turn the heat down to medium, cook for 2 minutes. Turn over and bring the heat back to high to sear the other side. Then cook for 2 minutes on medium heat. Drizzle with juice from 1/2 a lime. Cook for longer if you like it well done and for less time if it's fresh and you like it rare. Spoon the buttery lime sauce over the steaks while cooking.

Meanwhile, chop avocado and fresh coriander and season with a little sea salt and a tablespoon of lime juice. To plate, assemble some of the red peppers and tuna steaks with avocado salsa and more red peppers on top. Drizzle with extra lime juice and a little extra-virgin olive oil.

Look for Albacore or Skipjack tuna caught by pole, and avoid more vulnerable and threatened Bluefin tuna. Find pictures on Eat Drink Paleo website.

salmon fish cakes with radish & celery salsa

These are very popular in our home and with my readers. You can make a large batch and keep leftovers for lunch or as a post-workout snack. Salmon provides essential omega-3 fatty acids, while sweet potato is high in beta-carotene and vitamin C. Find pictures on Eat Drink Paleo website.

Preheat oven to 200°C (390°F). Bake sweet potato on a baking paper–lined tray for 30–40 minutes or until soft in the middle. Remove and cut in half to cool.

Meanwhile, boil some water in a pot. Add a few orange peels and the leftover celery stalk leaves. Place a colander or a sieve with salmon steaks inside over the pot and cover with a lid. Throw in the peas if they're frozen. Steam the fish for 2 minutes on each side or until light pink and just falling apart. You can also grill the salmon. Remove to a plate to cool down.

Peel the baked potato and mash it roughly with a fork or a potato masher. Remove the skin and bones from the salmon steaks, flake the flesh and mix with mashed potato, peas, spring onion, lemon zest, sea salt and pepper. Finally add the egg and tapioca flour and combine until well incorporated.

Heat coconut oil or ghee in a large frying pan until sizzling hot. Using a spoon, scoop a golf ball-sized amount of batter and use your fingers to slide the mixture off the spoon into the frying pan. Press and shape the batter into flat, round cakes. Don't overcrowd the pan and cook fish cakes in batches. Add extra oil when needed. Cook salmon cakes on medium-to-high heat for 4–5 minutes on each side, or until golden brown crusts form. While the salmon cakes are cooking, mix together the salsa ingredients in a bowl and set aside.

SERVES 3

For fish cakes

1 small sweet potato

Orange peel

2 salmon steaks

55g fresh or frozen baby peas

3 chopped spring onions

Zest from 1 lemon

2/3 tsp sea salt

Pinch of black pepper

1 egg

4 tbsp tapioca flour

2–3 tbsp ghee or coconut oil

For salsa

20 finely diced radishes

1 celery stick, finely diced (save celery stalk leaves)

2–3 spring onions, finely chopped

2 tbsp freshly squeezed orange juice (save orange peel)

2 tbsp lemon juice

1/2 tsp horseradish relish or grated horseradish

4 tbsp extra-virgin olive oil

2/3 tsp sea salt

garlic & saffron olive oil poached prawns salad

Inspired by the classic Spanish garlic prawns – the ones that sizzle in a clay dish at the table – this recipe uses a poaching method instead of applying high heat to olive oil, which retains all of its nutrients and delicate flavours and prevents oxidation. Find pictures on Eat Drink Paleo website.

SERVES 2

375ml extra-virgin olive oil

5 garlic cloves, sliced roughly

A few threads of saffron (powder can also be used)

salt

2 vines of cherry tomatoes (or use loose cherry tomatoes)

Olive oil

1–2 tbsp balsamic vinegar

12–14 fresh king prawns

For salad

Olive oil

1/2 long red chilli, finely chopped

Zest and juice of 1 lemon

2 medium courgettes, sliced in thin ribbons using a carrot peeler

1 tbsp fresh diced parsley

Sea salt and black pepper

Shaved aged Parmesan (optional)

Heat olive oil in a medium saucepan to 75–80°C (165°F), using a digital cooking thermometer. Add garlic, saffron, a pinch of salt and take off the heat. Stand aside to infuse for 30 minutes.

Preheat oven to 170°C (338°F). Place cherry tomatoes, still on the vine, on a roasting tray and drizzle with olive oil. Roast for 30 minutes. Then drizzle with balsamic vinegar and roast for a further 10 minutes. Set aside. Turn the oven down to 80°C (175°F).

Peel the prawns, removing the head but leaving the tail intact, and remove the dark vein from the back. Rinse and set aside. Prepare salad ingredients.

Place infused olive oil back on the heat and bring back to 75–80°C (175°F). Add prawns to a deep ovenproof dish and pour the oil with garlic over until prawns are submerged. Place uncovered dish in the oven for 10–15 minutes. Turn the prawns over after 5 minutes. The prawns will firm up and turn a light, pale yellow colour.

Meanwhile, heat a tablespoon of olive oil in a frying pan. Throw in chilli, lemon zest and courgette ribbons. Toss around for a minute to warm it up. In a salad bowl, combine courgette mixture with parsley, a pinch of salt and pepper, lemon juice and a little more extra-virgin olive oil. Toss through some cherry tomatoes and reserve the rest for plating. Gently remove the prawns and serve on top of the salad with roasted tomatoes and soft poached garlic.

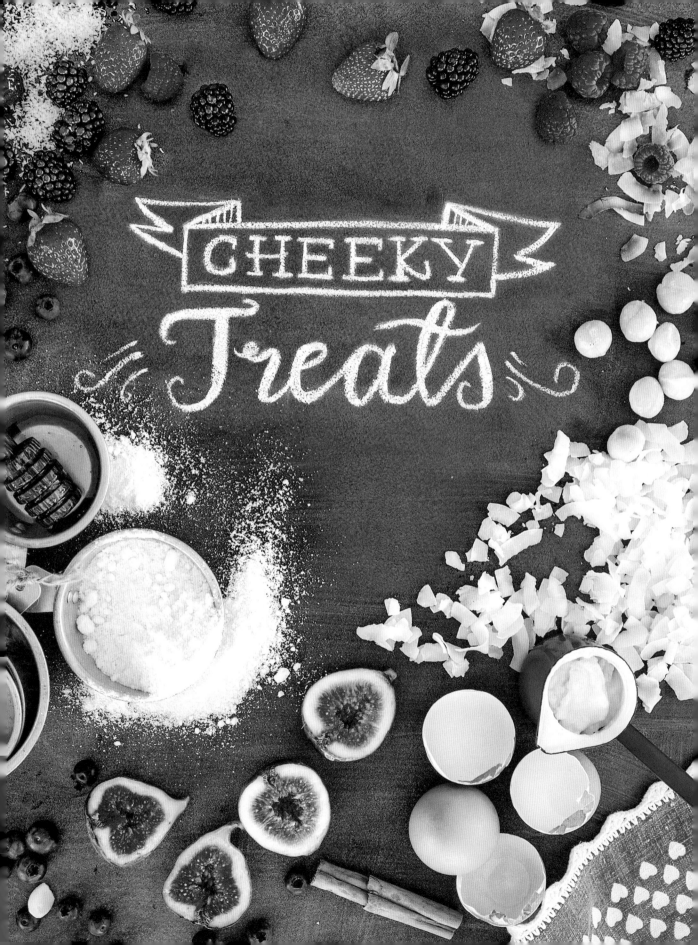

CHEEKY
Treats

chilli chocolate mousse

Whenever I offer this mousse to my guests I tell them it has no eggs or dairy and I dare them to guess what's in it. 'Avocado? No way!' they say in disbelief. 'How could something so rich and decadent actually be good for you?' Full of anti-inflammatory nutrients, antioxidants and healthy fats, this dessert is very easy to whip up even for the most unexpected dinner party.

SERVES 4

1 large ripe avocado, such as Hass

1 1/2 ripe bananas

6 tbsp raw cacao powder

3 tbsp coconut cream (from the top of the can)

1/2 vanilla pod, seeds scraped out

2 tbsp coconut sugar, honey or maple syrup

Pinch of sea salt

1/2 tsp red chilli flakes

Optional

Dark chocolate flakes, raspberries and chilli flakes for garnish

Cut avocado in half and remove the stone. Scoop out the flesh and add to a food processor or blender together with chopped banana and cacao powder. Whizz up until smooth.

Transfer to a large bowl, add cream, vanilla seeds and your choice of sweetener. Whisk using an electric blender until well combined, fluffy and smooth. Fold in salt and chilli flakes.

You can serve right away but it's best to refrigerate the mousse to set for around 1 hour. You can set it in ramekins or small serving glasses. Garnish with dark chocolate flakes, raspberries and a little extra sprinkle of chilli flakes.

Raw cacao powder has more antioxidants than blueberries, red wine or green tea. You can replace raw cacao powder with melted dark chocolate and, if looking for a lower carbohydrate version, replace some of the banana with extra avocado and coconut cream.

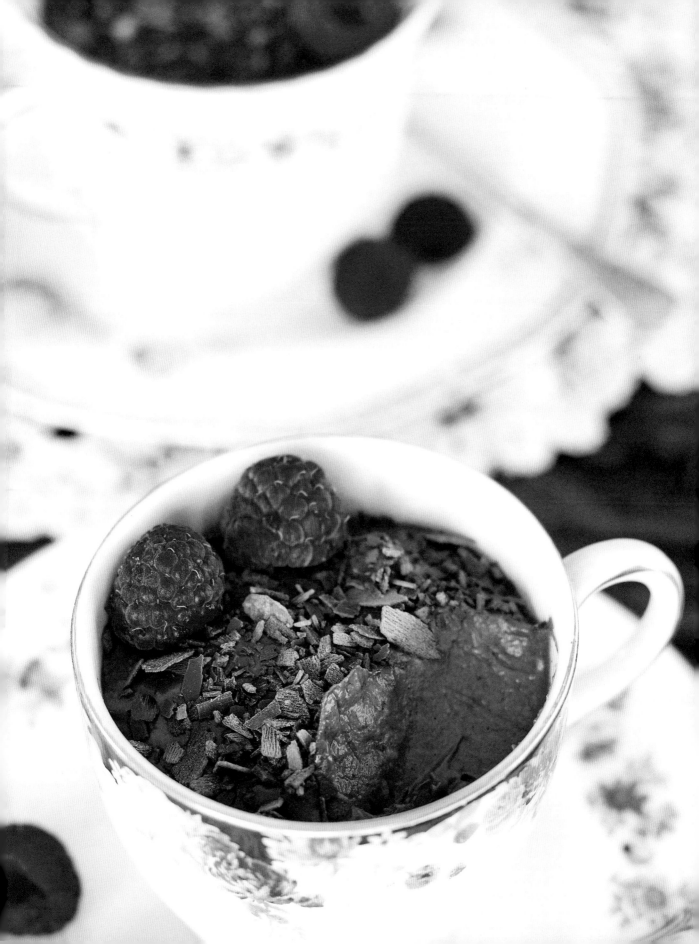

macadamia cakies

These look and taste like macadamia cookies but the texture is a little more moist and soft due to almond meal. Basically, they're little cakes pretending to be cookies. No point calling them what they're not, so from now on they are known as 'cakies'.

MAKES ABOUT 12-15 CAKIES

275–375g raw macadamia nuts

2 eggs

5 tbsp coconut oil, melted

3 tbsp raw honey

1 tbsp vanilla extract

150g almond meal

2 1/2 tbsp tapioca flour

3/4 tsp cinnamon powder

Pinch of salt

1/3 tsp gluten-free baking powder

Preheat oven to 180°C (355°F). Chop most of the macadamia nuts into smaller pieces, or place them in a plastic bag and whack a few times with a rolling pin. Reserve some for decoration. Place in a bowl.

Whisk liquid ingredients in a bowl. Add almond meal, tapioca, cinnamon powder, salt and sprinkle baking powder. Fold until well incorporated. Add the macadamia nuts to the mix and stir through. Refrigerate for 5 minutes.

Make a piping bag or a cone out of baking paper. I use a sandwich bag with one of the bottom corners chopped off. Scoop the cake mixture into the piping bag. Line a flat tray with a double sheet of baking paper and squeeze small dollops (large walnut size) of cake mix, 2cm apart. Stick a few remaining macadamia nuts on top and use your fingers or a spatula to flatten the cakes a little.

Bake for 15 minutes. Remove and set aside for 5–10 minutes to cool down before serving. Keep in an airtight container in a cool place for up to 3–4 days.

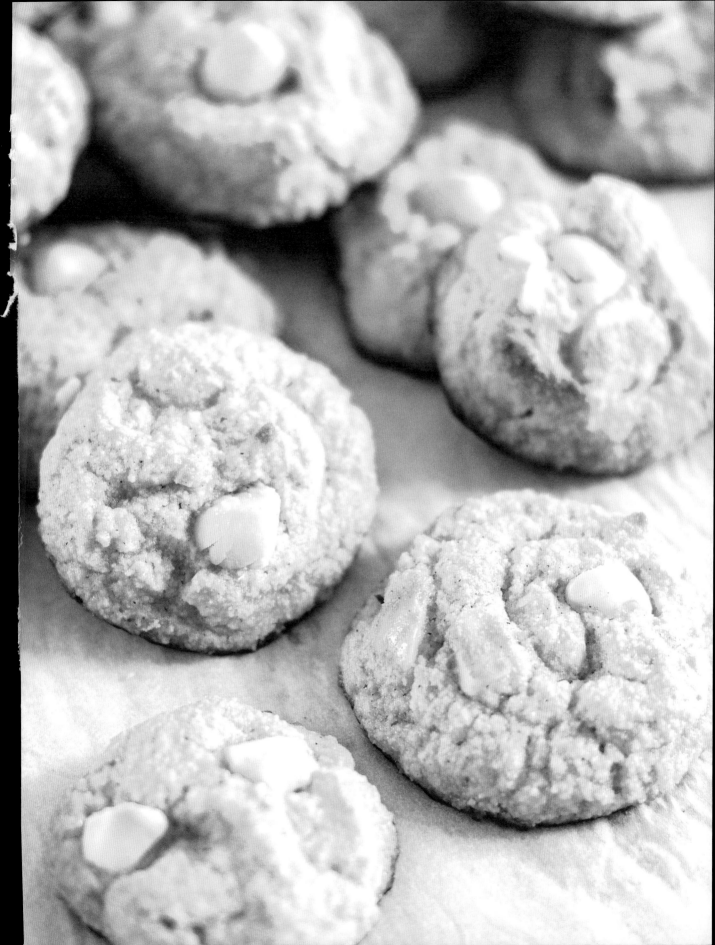

raspberry & honey chocolate torte

Full of antioxidants – found in raw cacao and fresh raspberries – and the healthy saturated fat of coconut oil, you won't feel guilty indulging in this scrumptious chocolate cake. It does have a fair amount of almond meal, which is on the higher end of omega-6 fatty acids content, as well as honey, so leave it for special occasions.

  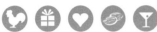

SERVES 10

185ml coconut oil (melted)

60g raw cacao powder (you can use baking cocoa powder too)

185ml raw honey

30ml port or dry sherry

125ml water

4 eggs (yolks and whites separated)

220g almond meal

65g raspberries (defrosted or fresh)

1 tsp gluten–free baking powder

Pinch of sea salt

Fresh raspberries & desiccated coconut to garnish

> You can replace raw cacao powder with melted dark chocolate and use green leaf stevia or coconut syrup instead of honey. Just adjust the amount based on the concentration of the sweetener.

Preheat oven to 170°C (338°F). Brush a round 22cm cake tin with melted coconut oil to lightly grease, and line the base and sides with non-stick baking paper.

Combine cacao powder, honey, coconut oil, port and water in a bowl and whisk together until incorporated.

In a different bowl, whisk the egg yolks for a few minutes until thick and glossy. Fold in the chocolate mixture and almond meal and raspberries. Sift or sprinkle the baking powder over the mixture rather than dropping it in one spot to ensure uniformity.

Use an electric beater to whisk egg whites with a little pinch of salt in a clean dry bowl until soft peaks form. Use a spoon to fold some of the egg whites into chocolate mixture until combined. Gently fold in remaining egg whites until just combined.

Pour mixture into the prepared cake tin. Bake for 40 minutes or until a skewer inserted into the centre comes out clean. Set aside in the pan to cool completely.

Once cool, remove the cake onto a serving plate and garnish with fresh raspberries and desiccated coconut. Serve with a generous side of coconut cream or regular double cream.

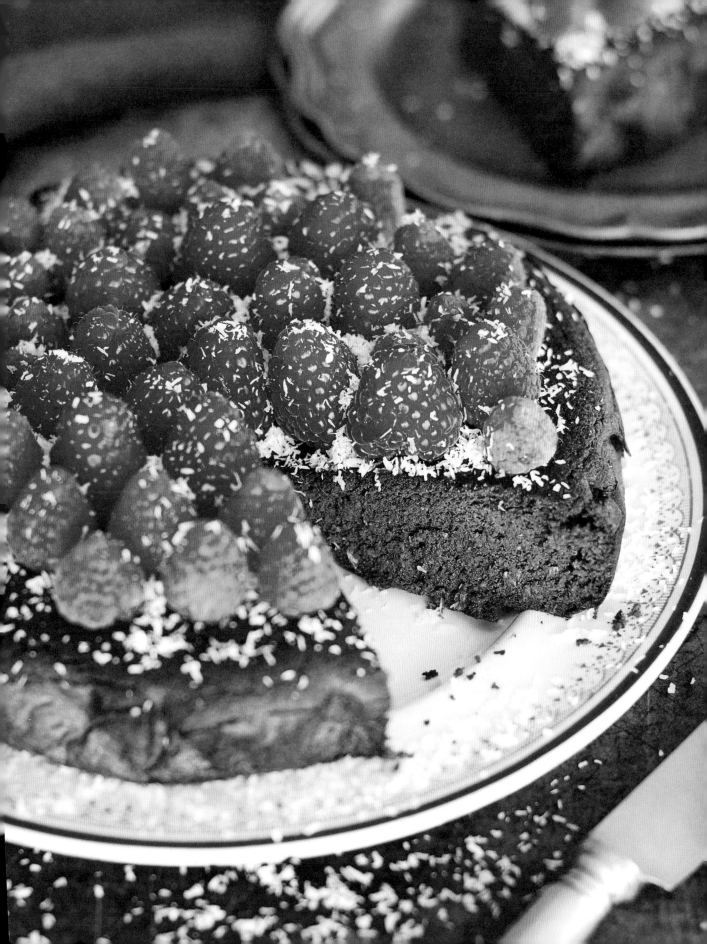

ricotta cheesecake with grilled peaches

If heaven exists and it's up in the clouds, this is the cake they serve for afternoon tea – fluffy, light and subtle textures with flavours of tangy, juicy peaches peeking through like rays of sunshine. This cheesecake is high in protein, calcium and vitamin C; and ricotta is a cheese primarily made from whey, which is less problematic than cheeses that contain mostly casein protein. However, if you're avoiding all dairy, you'll have to sit this one out. More for me!

SERVES 8

A little melted coconut oil

650g fresh ricotta cheese

7 tbsp green leaf stevia powder

1 tbsp tapioca flour (or similar starch such as potato)

1 tsp vanilla extract or fresh vanilla seeds from the pod

4 eggs (yolks and whites separated)

5 tbsp coconut cream (from the top of the can, avoid the water)

3–4 large ripe peaches

1–2 tbsp coconut sugar

1 tbsp cinnamon powder

A few leaves of fresh basil

> You can use a different type of sweetener instead of stevia, such as coconut syrup or honey, although it might change the colour of the cake. Any other fruit can be used instead of peaches – fresh berries, kiwifruit, mango and even fresh figs drizzled with a little honey and lemon.

Preheat oven to 160°C (320°F). Brush a round 22cm cake tin with melted coconut oil to lightly grease, and line the base and sides with non-stick baking paper.

Beat together the ricotta, stevia powder, tapioca, vanilla, egg yolks and coconut cream. In a separate clean bowl, beat the egg whites until stiff peaks form, then fold into the ricotta mixture. Pour into the cake tin and bake for 50–60 minutes until golden brown on top.

Meanwhile, remove stones from the peaches and cut them into even wedges. Place on a greased flat baking tray on top of baking paper. Sprinkle with coconut sugar and cinnamon. Place the tray with the peaches on the lower shelf of the oven about half way through cheesecake baking.

Remove the cake from the oven and set aside to cool; it will sink slightly. Place the tray with peaches under a medium grill to brown and caramelise the tops for a further 10 minutes or so.

Starting in the middle, place the grilled peaches on top of the cheesecake in a snail shape. Garnish with fresh berries and fresh basil.

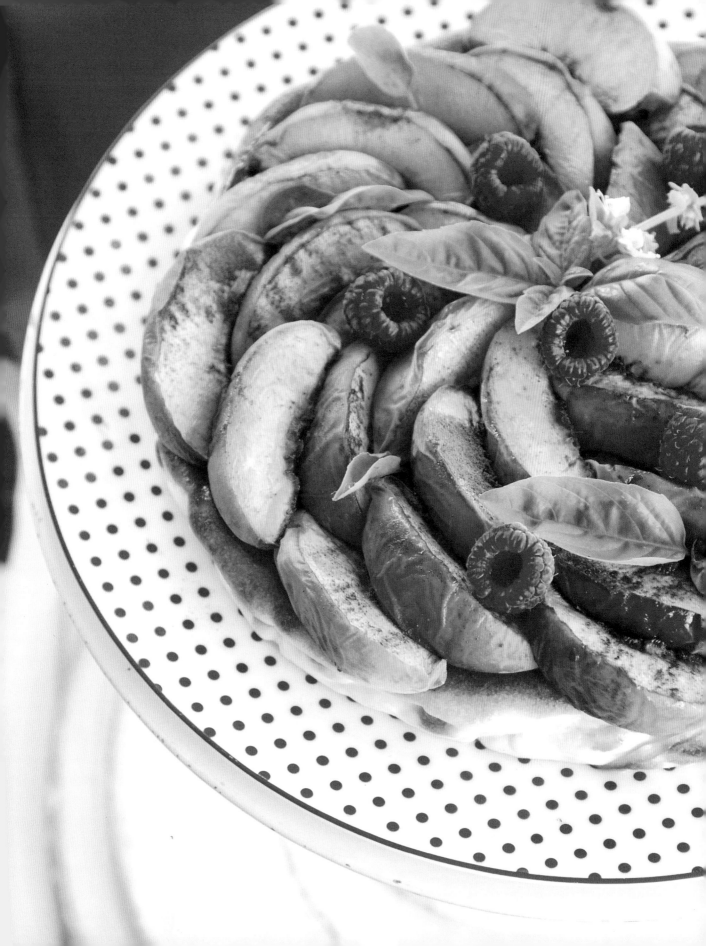

mango & blackberry meringue roulade

Take awesome stuff and roll it inside more awesome stuff and this is what you get. My paleo take on the classic meringue roulade was a real crowd pleaser the first time I made it. It's easy to make and the best part is you can really play with the fillings. How about strawberries and melted dark chocolate or peaches and toasted almond flakes with some Amaretto liqueur whisked into the cream?

SERVES 6

For the meringue

5 egg whites

Pinch of salt

6 tsp green leaf stevia powder

2 tsp tapioca flour

2 tsp white wine vinegar or apple cider vinegar

1 tsp vanilla extract

For the filling

50g desiccated or grated coconut, plus coconut flakes

375ml coconut cream (about a can)

4 tbsp double cream (if not using dairy, use an extra can of coconut cream)

2–3 tsp stevia or other preferred natural sweetener

1 mango, diced

130g blackberries or other berries

Mango and berries to garnish

Preheat oven to 160°C (320°F). Grease and line a flat baking tray with non-stick baking paper.

Beat egg whites with a pinch of salt to soft peaks and add the stevia powder, one teaspoon at a time, until well incorporated. Add tapioca, white wine vinegar and vanilla extract, and whisk together until combined.

Spoon the mixture evenly onto the baking tray and smooth the top. Try to maintain a square or rectangular shape that is wide enough to roll into a log. Bake for 20–25 minutes or until light golden and firm. Cool completely.

Roast coconut flakes in the oven at 160°C (320°F) for about 2 minutes or until golden brown. Lay a piece of fresh greaseproof paper out and flip the meringue over onto it, carefully pull away the used paper and discard.

Remove the thickened part of the coconut cream from the can to a bowl. Whisk with double cream together with the stevia or other preferred sweetener. Spread the cream over the meringue surface, keeping it close to the middle. Cover with half the mango, blackberries, and some roasted coconut flakes. Roll the meringue up lengthways using the paper to help turn it over. Secure with some plastic wrap and place in the fridge for 30 minutes to an hour. Serve sprinkled with coconut and remaining mango and berries.

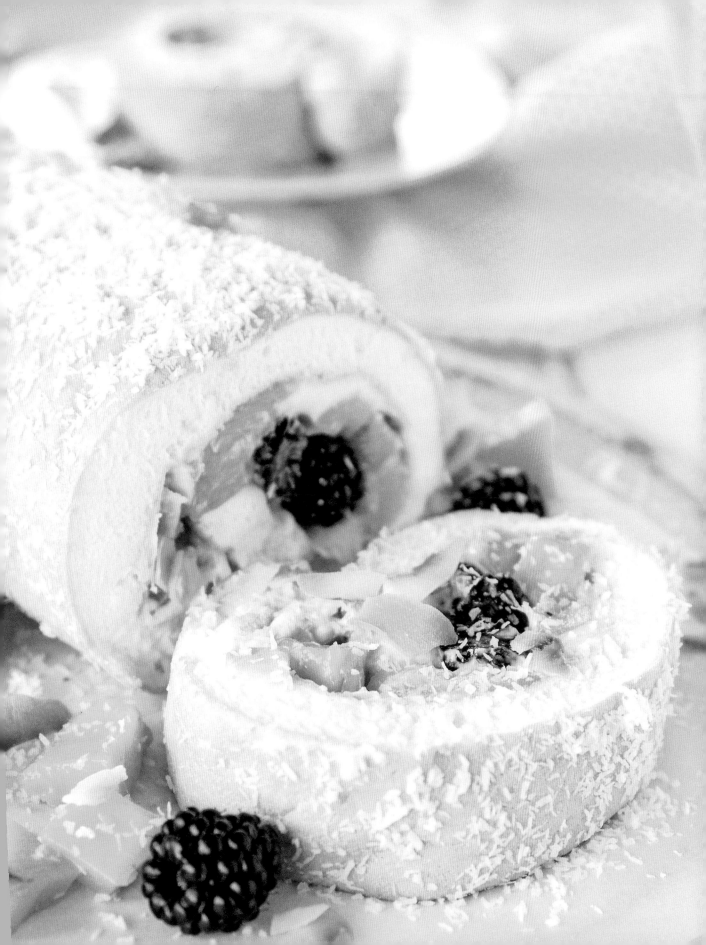

banana muffins with strawberry butter

Believe me when I say that these taste and smell more delicious than what you're imagining in your head right now. The muffins will last a few days and make an easy addition to kids' lunch boxes. You can use normal butter but my super-easy strawberry version is to die for and really adds that little bit of decadence to the treat.

SERVES 6–8

A little coconut or olive oil

110g almond meal

50g coconut flour

50g tapioca flour

2 tsp baking powder

1/4 tsp bicarbonate of soda

1 1/2 ripe bananas, mashed

1 tsp cinnamon powder

Pinch of nutmeg

1 egg

125ml coconut milk

3 tbsp raw honey

1/2 vanilla pod, seeds scraped out (or use 1 tsp of vanilla extract)

1/2 banana, sliced

120g strawberry butter (page 194)

Preheat oven to 200°C (390°F) and pre-grease the muffin tin/s with some coconut or olive oil.

Combine almond meal, flours, baking powder and bicarbonate of soda and mix until well incorporated. Add the mashed banana, cinnamon, nutmeg, egg, coconut milk, honey and vanilla seeds and process together using an electric mixer. Finally, fold in sliced banana.

Divide the mixture between muffin tray casings. Bake for 15–17 minutes, or until raised and brown on the top. Serve with strawberry butter on top.

This recipe can be done without eggs, just add a little more coconut milk instead. These will keep well in an airtight container or you can wrap them individually in some plastic wrap and keep in the fridge for lunches and afternoon snacks.

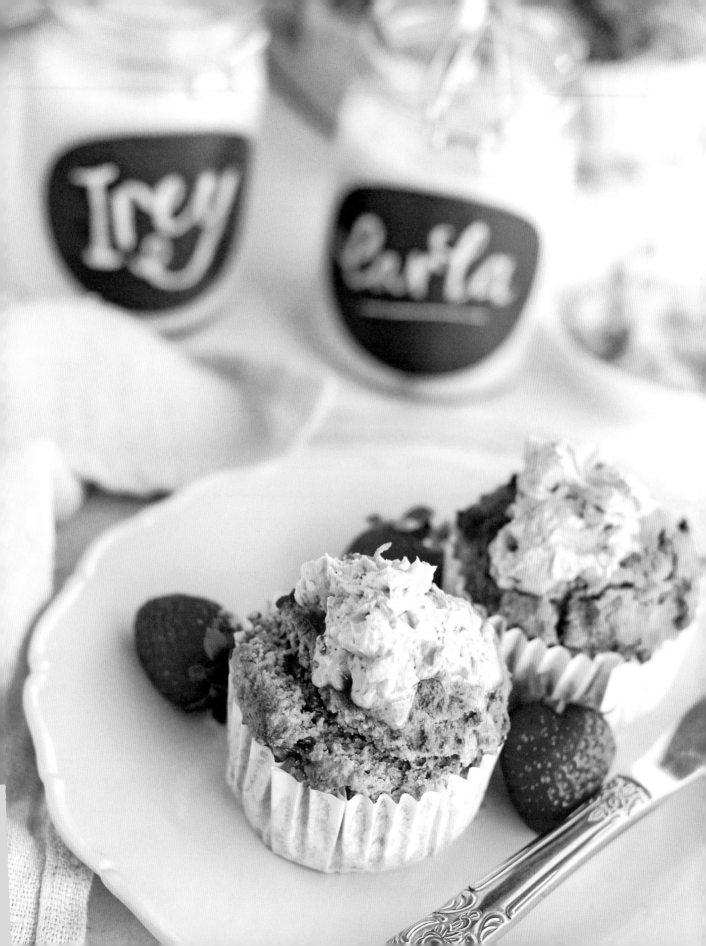

blood orange & strawberry granita

Originating from Italy, granita is a semi-frozen dessert that can easily be made at home. Once you know the basic method and ratios, you can create new flavour combinations using freshly squeezed fruit juices, infused teas and coffee, and with coconut milk for a creamier effect. You can even make savoury versions with tomato, carrot and beetroot juices.

SERVES 3–4

Juice of 3 blood oranges, plus zest of one of them

10 medium strawberries, leaves removed

300ml water

Juice of 1/2 lime, about 1 tbsp

1 tbsp green leaf stevia powder

Dash of vanilla extract or fresh vanilla seeds

Extra strawberries and a blood orange for garnish

Combine all ingredients in a saucepan and bring to boil. Simmer for 2–3 minutes, take off the stove and allow to cool to room temperature.

Process mixture in a blender and pour into a shallow tray. Cover with plastic wrap and place in the freezer until solidified. Once frozen, remove from the freezer and let it thaw just a little before scraping the ice with a fork. Serve the shaved granita ice in glasses. Garnish with strawberries and blood orange slices.

You can use normal orange juice instead of blood orange.

Other granita combinations

Apple juice, lime juice and fresh mint

Amaretto liqueur and lemon juice

Tomato, lemon, chilli and sea salt

Blueberry, beetroot and basil

Carrot, ginger, lemon and honey

Black coffee, vanilla and maple syrup

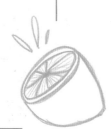

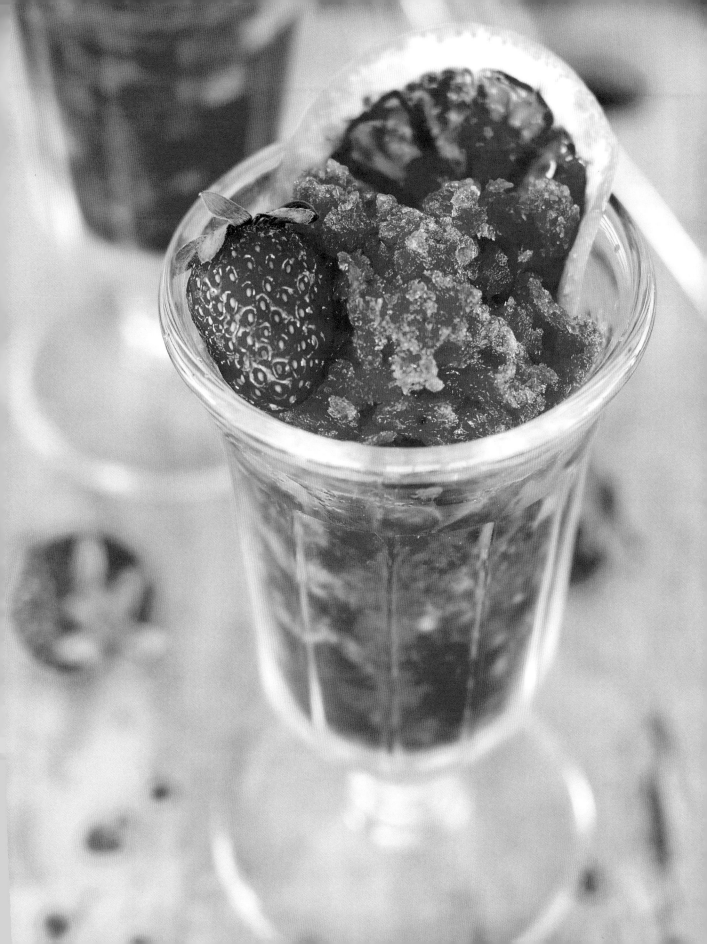

double-decker lamingtons

This is a paleo-friendly version of a classic Australian lamington. These look, smell and taste like the real thing except that the texture is a little denser and more moist, rather than fluffy and dry. Visit the website for more detailed pictures of how to make these little beauties.

MAKES 16 SQUARES

For the sponge cake

160ml coconut oil

4 tbsp raw honey or 2 1/2 tbsp green leaf stevia powder

1 tsp vanilla extract

3 whole eggs

1 tsp gluten-free baking powder or bicarbonate of soda

50g tapioca flour

75g almond meal

For the chocolate and coconut icing

160ml coconut oil

60g cocoa powder

1 tsp vanilla extract

3 tbsp coconut or almond milk

2 tbsp maple syrup or 1 tbsp green leaf stevia powder

165g desiccated coconut (unsweetened)

Preheat oven to 165°C (330°F). Grease a 2cm deep, 20cm x 30cm base baking tray with olive oil. Line with baking paper.

Dissolve coconut oil, honey and vanilla extract and whisk together until well incorporated.

Using an electric mixer, beat eggs for 5 minutes until thick and foamy. Gradually add coconut oil mix while beating the eggs. Add baking powder, tapioca flour and almond meal. Using a whisk or a spatula, fold for 10–15 seconds until incorporated.

Pour mixture into the prepared tray. Bake for 20 minutes or until a skewer inserted into the centre comes out clean. Turn the sponge cake onto a wire rack and set aside to cool completely. When cooled, trim the edges off and cut into four equal strips.

To make chocolate icing, combine coconut oil, cocoa, vanilla, coconut milk and syrup in a bowl. Whisk for 1 minute. Spread desiccated coconut on a separate plate.

Spread a thin layer of chocolate icing on one side of the sponge cake strips. Stick two strips into one, chocolate sides in. Cut strips into equal lamington pieces.

Using two forks, dip and coat lamington pieces with a thin layer of chocolate icing and then dip and roll in coconut. Set aside on a wire rack for 1–2 hours before serving. If the icing starts to set while coating, add 1–2 tablespoons of hot water and whisk through again.

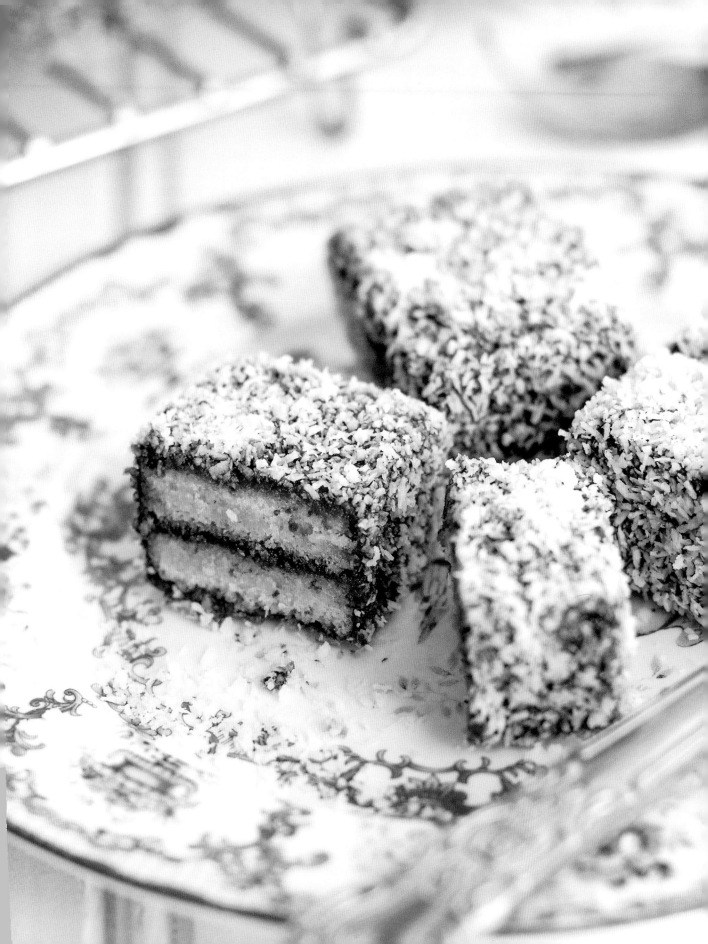

cherry macaroons

There are macarons – the French kind, glossy, perfectly shaped almond biscuits with exquisite creamy filling; and then there are macaroons – chewy, rough around the edges, coconut domes many of us associated with childhood trips to the local bakery. Both are made with egg whites as a base, both are very tasty, but one of them follows a complex recipe with multiple processes that requires time, patience and a little skill. This is the easy option!

MAKES 16 MACAROONS

A little olive oil

3 egg whites

Pinch of salt

Pinch of cream of tartar

A few drops of white vinegar

2 tbsp coconut syrup or other natural sweetener

1 tsp rose water

55g almond meal

165g grated or desiccated coconut, unsweetened

75g pitted cherries, roughly chopped

Preheat oven to 170°C (338°F). Grease a flat oven tray with a little olive oil and line with baking paper.

Beat egg whites with a pinch of salt until soft peaks form, then add cream of tartar, vinegar, coconut syrup and rose water. Beat until glossy and fold in almond meal, shredded coconut and cherries until well incorporated. Using a teaspoon and your fingers, scoop walnut-sized dollops of mixture on to a baking tray, at least 1cm apart. Bake for 15–17 minutes until raised and golden brown. Cool down before eating.

> Cream of tartar is a byproduct from wine making, also known as potassium hydrogen tartrate. It's an acidic white powder used in conjunction with baking soda as a raising agent in baking or to increase the stability and volume of beaten egg whites. White vinegar can also be used. You can use fresh or canned pitted cherries, look for unsweetened varieties. Rose water can be purchased in the baking section of your supermarket or can be omitted if you don't like the rose-petal flavour, even if it's just a hint.

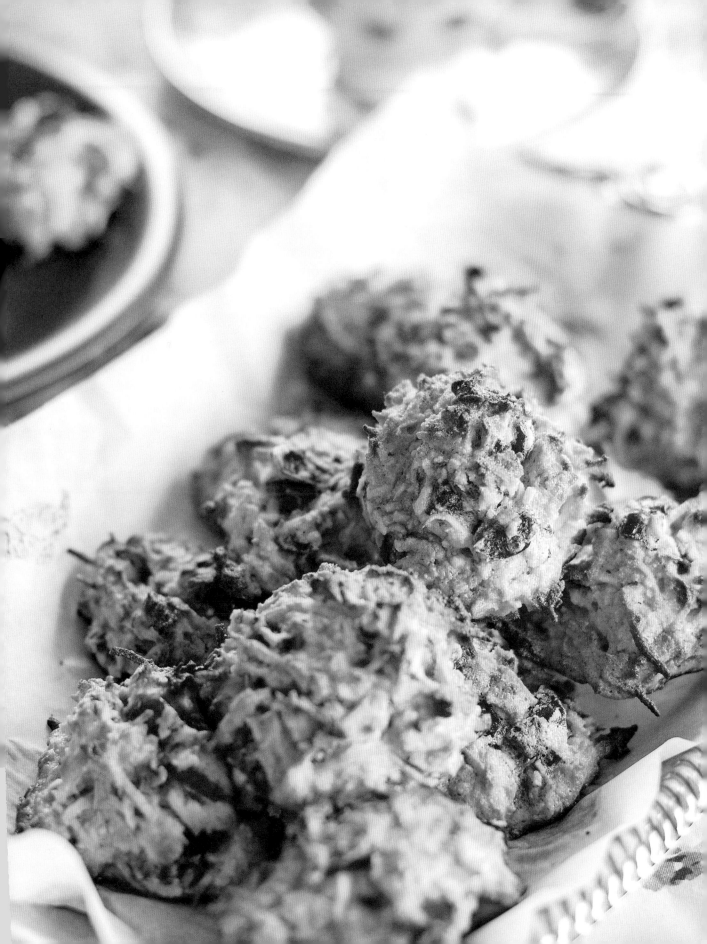

spiced stewed rhubarb

This is a very quick and easy dessert packed with vitamin C and calcium from the rhubarb and yoghurt. Those avoiding dairy can serve the rhubarb with nuts and some coconut cream or coconut yoghurt.

SERVES 4–5

250g diced rhubarb (about 1 bunch of rhubarb)

120g diced ripe pineapple

Juice of 1 orange

1/2 tsp Chinese five-spice powder

2 tbsp raw honey

30ml water

To serve

8 tbsp natural, full-fat Greek yoghurt

4 tbsp toasted flaked almonds

Combine ingredients in a saucepan, bring to simmer and turn the heat to low. Cook on low heat for 10–15 minutes until soft. Serve warm with some yoghurt and toasted almonds or other nuts.

You can pre-toast flaked almonds in a dry frying pan or in the oven on 160°C (320°F) for about 5 minutes.

Learn how to make a dairy-free coconut yoghurt on page 182.

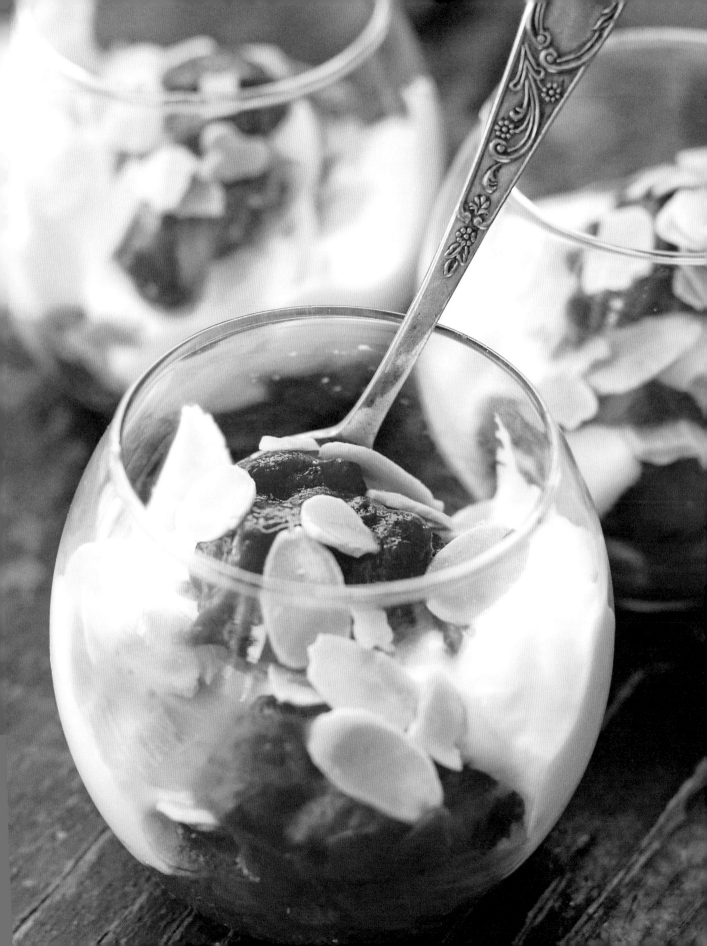

jaffa rum balls

These wickedly delicious rum balls are a perfect little treat minus the guilt. They're great to keep on hand as a quick energy snack or to pack as part of your lunch. In addition, they are super easy to make – there's absolutely no cooking involved – and your kids can help to roll the balls.

MAKES 20 BALLS

110g almond or hazelnut meal

30ml dark rum

6 tbsp coconut oil

3 tbsp cocoa powder

2 tbsp maple syrup or honey

100g sultanas

Zest of 2 oranges

55g desiccated coconut

Extra cocoa and desiccated coconut

Place all ingredients in a food processor. Purée and blend everything into a thick, doughy mixture. It should stick together as it comes off the sides.

Roll into small balls using your fingers. Coconut oil in the mixture will keep your hands greasy and the mixture won't stick. Dust the finished balls with desiccated coconut and extra cocoa powder. Place on a plate, cover with plastic wrap and refrigerate. Store in a cool place, fridge if possible, before serving.

View pictures on Eat Drink Paleo website.

no-bake energy balls

MAKES 8–10 BALLS

70g almonds

70g brazil nuts

500ml water

1 tbsp lemon juice

75g sunflower seeds

1 tsp orange or lemon zest

1 tsp vanilla extract

5–6 dates, chopped

1 1/2 tbsp raw cacao powder

1 1/2 tbsp raw honey

2 tbsp coconut oil

1 tbsp chia seeds

Place almonds and brazil nuts in water with a tablespoon of lemon and soak for 4–6 hours. This will remove some of the phytic acid and activate the nuts, making them easier to digest. Rinse well and remove the skin from the almonds unless using blanched nuts. The skin should come off easily.

Place soaked nuts with the rest of ingredients, except for chia seeds, in a food processor. Process until thick batter is formed. Transfer to a bowl and mix with chia seeds. Roll heaped tablespoon amounts of dough into balls in between your hands and transfer to a sealed container. Refrigerate for a couple of hours to set.

These will keep in the fridge for up to a week. You can roll them in extra desiccated coconut or dust with extra raw cacao powder.

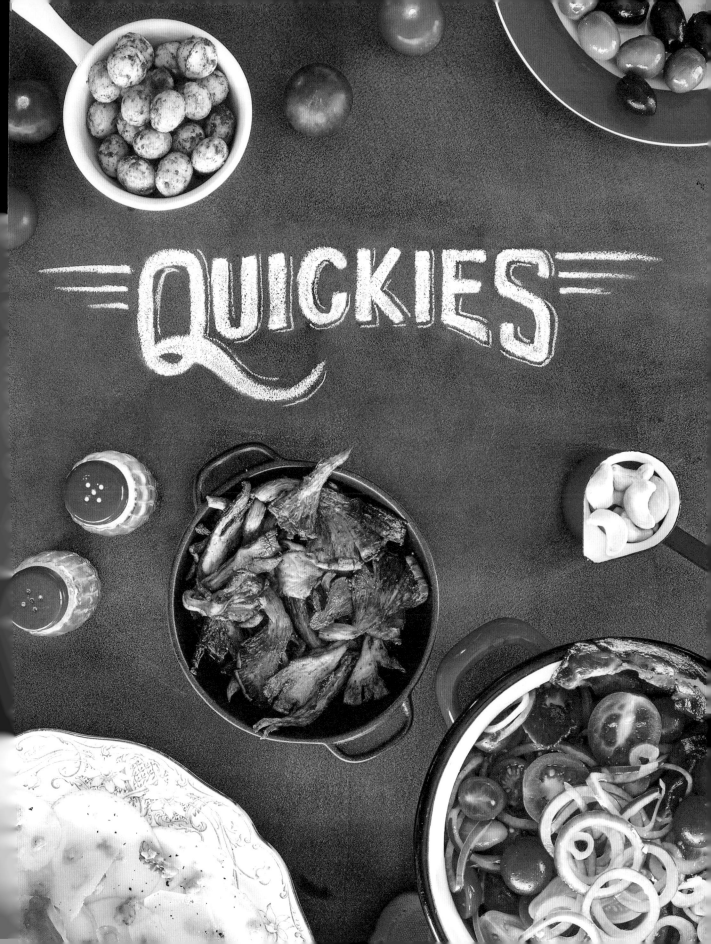

QUICKIES

kedgeree devilled eggs

This recipe is inspired by Kedgeree, a traditional British breakfast from colonial India, which you can often find in cafes these days. It's usually made with rice, smoked fish, boiled eggs, curry powder and herbs. I took away the rice and came up with these little beauties.

MAKES 10–12 HALVES

6 eggs

1/3 whole smoked trout (medium size) or 1 smoked trout fillet

3 tbsp coconut oil

1/2 brown onion, chopped

1 tsp ghee

1 tsp curry powder

1 tbsp lemon juice

2 tbsp mayonnaise

Pinch of salt and pepper

Some fresh dill to serve

You can purchase a whole smoked trout from most fishmongers and supermarkets. Use trout leftovers in a salad, with scrambled eggs or in a celeriac remoulade. Covered with some plastic wrap or in an airtight container, devilled eggs will keep in the fridge for a few days. They make a good addition to a lunch box or you can eat them as a snack.

Bring a medium saucepan of water to rapid boil. Gently lower eggs and swirl them around gently so that yolks don't set too close to one side of the shell. Cook for 10–12 minutes until hard-boiled. Strain and submerge in cold water.

Peel the skin off the trout and remove the thicker parts of the flesh, enough to fit in a palm. Pick out the bones and break into small flakes. Heat coconut oil in a medium frying pan and cook the trout flesh for 5–7 minutes, breaking it into small pieces, until very crisp and golden brown. Drain on some paper towel.

Sauté onion in ghee, on medium heat, for about 8 minutes, until softened and golden. Add curry powder and stir through. Remove to a bowl.

Peel boiled eggs carefully. Cut in halves, lengthways, and remove the yolks, transferring into a bowl. Mix the yolks with curried onion, 2 tablespoons of fried trout, lemon juice, 1 teaspoon of mayonnaise and a pinch of salt and pepper.

Fill the egg white halves with yolk mixture and top up with a little dollop of mayonnaise, some fried smoked trout and fresh dill.

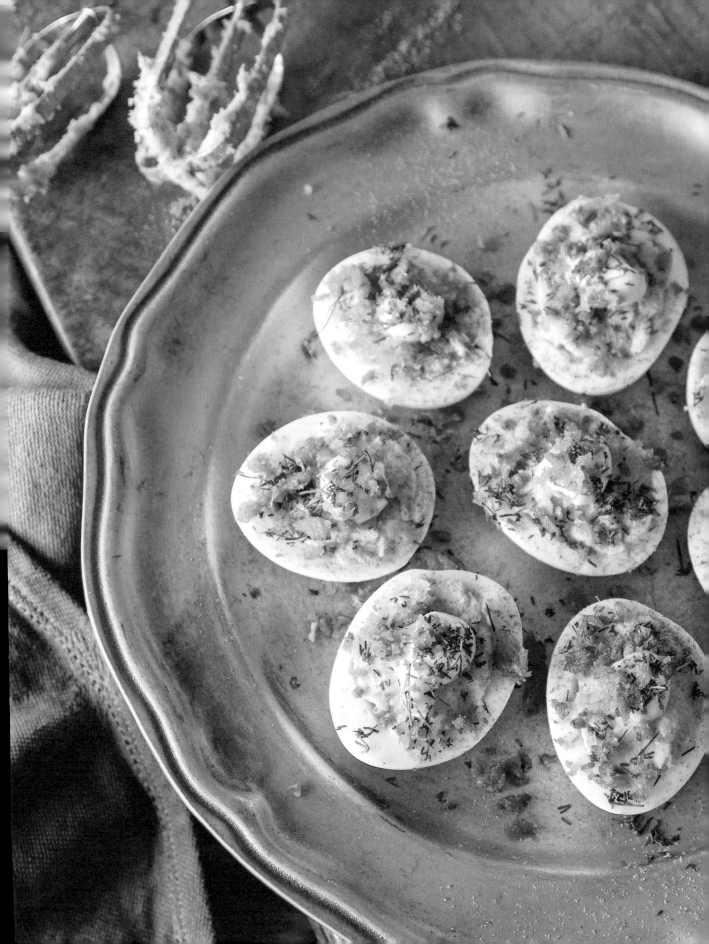

pear & walnut carpaccio

Walnut and pear go beautifully together, even when served as a semi-savoury dish. Pecorino is a cheese made with sheep's milk and is often a good option for those sensitive to cow's milk dairy. It is completely optional but it does add a nice touch of saltiness to balance out the sweetness of the pear.

SERVES 2 AS A STARTER

2 Williams pears (ripe but not too soft)

1/4 lemon

A few shavings of Pecorino (sheep's milk cheese)

Wild rocket or mustard leaves

A few walnuts, broken up

Lemon juice

Extra-virgin olive oil

Walnut dressing

4–5 walnuts

1 small garlic clove

2 tbsp macadamia oil or extra-virgin olive oil

1 tbsp white wine vinegar

Pinch of sea salt

Slice pear into paper-thin slivers and drizzle and rub with a little lemon to prevent browning. Arrange on a large, flat platter.

Grind walnuts and garlic using a mortar and pestle and mix with macadamia oil, vinegar and salt. Drizzle over pear and sprinkle with a few walnuts. Serve with a bunch of wild rocket drizzled with lemon and some extra-virgin olive oil.

Wild rocket or mustard leaves have a lovely peppery flavour but normal rocket or green spinach can also be used.

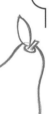

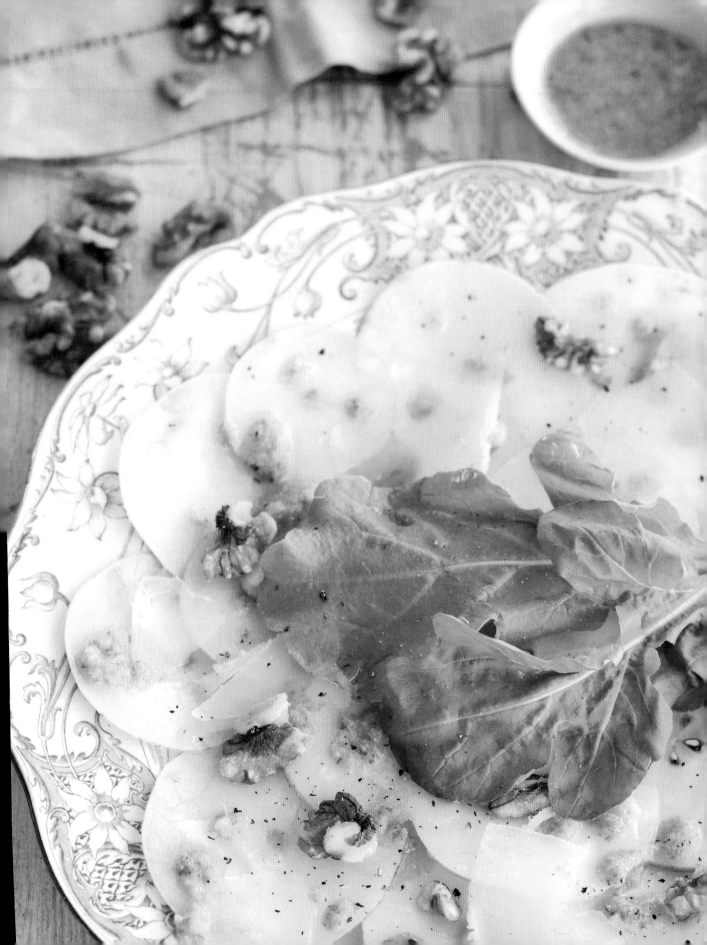

spinach tahini dip

MAKES 250ML

1 tbsp extra-virgin olive oil

1 large bunch of spinach, chopped

2 garlic cloves, peeled and roughly chopped

2 tbsp lemon juice

2 1/2 tbsp tahini

35g macadamia nuts

2/3 tsp salt

Pinch of black pepper

Heat a small saucepan with olive oil. Add spinach and chopped garlic, cook for a minute or two, until spinach is soft and wilted. Remove to a plate and drizzle with lemon juice. Once cooled down, add to a food processor and mix with tahini, macadamia nuts, salt and pepper until smooth. Eat with vegetable crudités or serve as a condiment with some seafood or chicken.

spicy kale chips

Kale chips are the popcorn of the paleo world. Kale is ridiculously nutritious – lots of iron, calcium and vitamin C - and it's really easy to make crispy chips with. Make sure to consume kale chips soon after they're ready or they will lose their crispiness. Omit paprika if avoiding nightshades.

SERVES 2

10 kale leaves (on a stalk)

1 1/2 tbsp virgin olive oil

1 tsp paprika

1/2 tsp coriander seed powder

2/3 tsp ground cumin powder

1 tsp sea salt

Preheat oven to 170°C (350°F).

Pull kale leaves away from the stalks and cut into 2–3cm pieces with scissors, or tear with your hands. Wash and dry the leaves in a salad spinner or pat dry with some paper towel. Toss clean leaves with olive oil, spices and sea salt.

Scatter in a large oven tray and bake for 15 minutes, tossing them around every 5 minutes to prevent burning and to make sure they dry out and roast evenly on all sides. Kale chips may be ready in 12 minutes depending on your oven and the amount of leaves you can fit in your tray. You can bake them in batches.

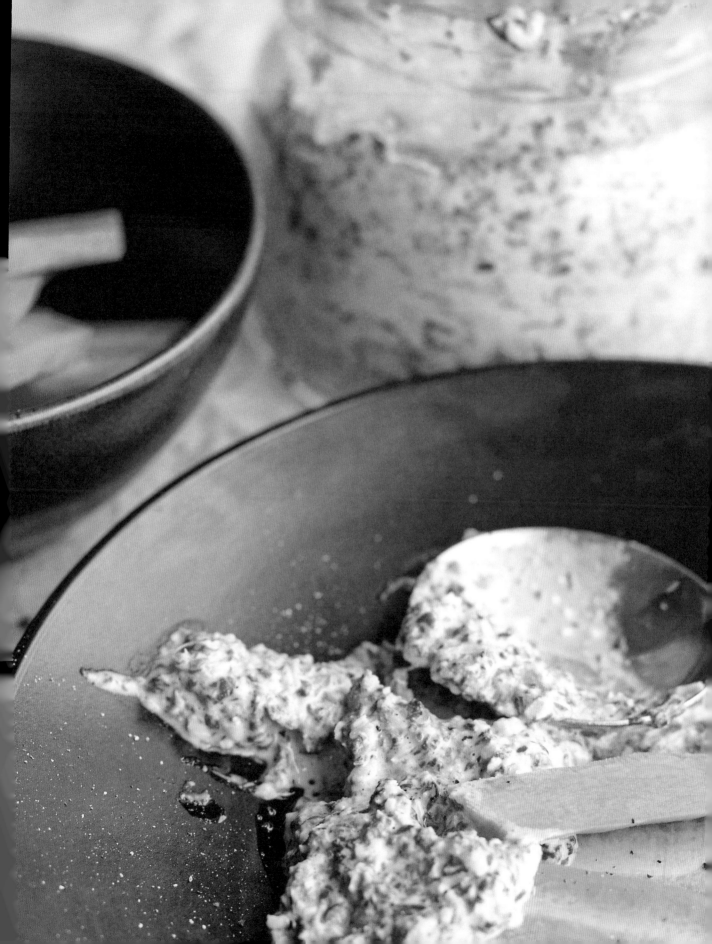

roasted cauliflower popcorn

SERVES 2–4 AS A SNACK

3 tbsp virgin olive oil

2 garlic cloves, finely chopped

1/2 long red chilli, finely chopped

1/2 tsp turmeric powder

2/3 tsp garlic powder

1/2 tsp paprika

1/2 tsp coriander seed powder

2 tbsp red wine vinegar

1 cauliflower head, cut into small florets

Preheat oven to 180°C (355°F). Mix all ingredients in a bowl, add cauliflower florets and toss until well covered. Spread evenly in a large roasting tray and bake in the oven for 25–30 minutes or until lightly browned, stirring at half way.

prosciutto-wrapped asparagus

MAKES 12

6 prosciutto strips, halved lengthways

12 asparagus spears, washed and ends trimmed

Ghee for frying

Place one prosciutto strip on a chopping board at a 45° angle. Place one of the asparagus spears on top of the meat, perpendicular to it. The tip of the asparagus should be lined up with the bottom of the prosciutto strip. Wrap the bottom end of prosciutto over the asparagus and, holding the meat tight, start rolling the asparagus up. The prosciutto strip will wrap around the whole length of the spear because it's on an angle. Don't worry if parts of the asparagus spears are not covered completely. Repeat with the remaining asparagus and prosciutto.

Heat some ghee in a large, flat frying pan to sizzling hot. Fry wrapped asparagus spears for 1–2 minutes on each side or until prosciutto is brown and crispy.

Find pictures on Eat Drink Paleo website.

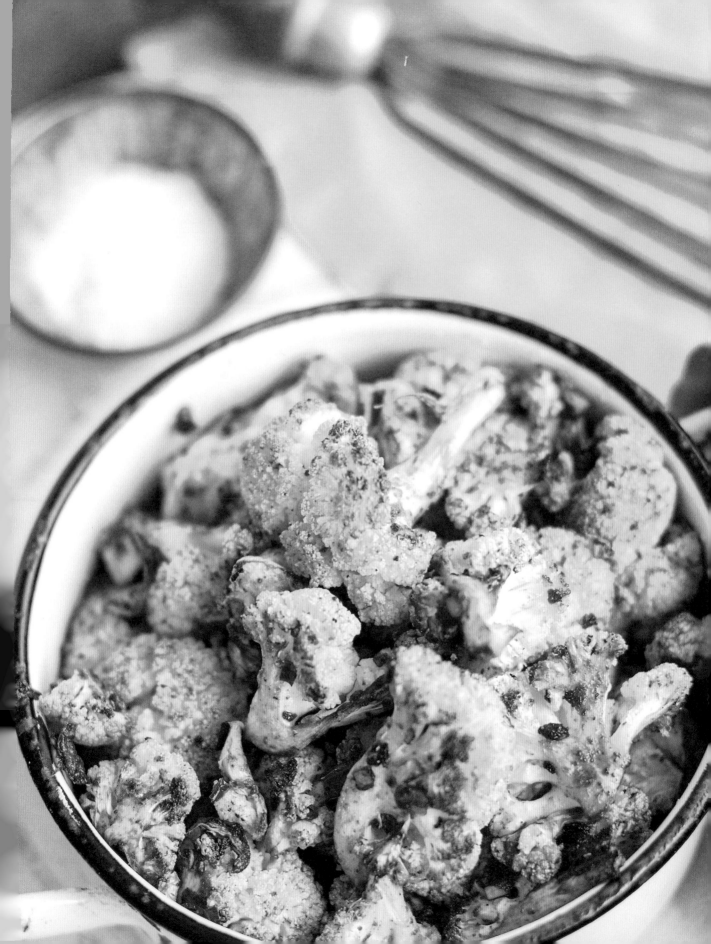

smoky oyster mushrooms

These smoky flavoured oyster mushrooms are quite meaty and have a gorgeous savoury umami flavour (which basically means they taste freaking amazing). Eat as chips or add to the top of salads, stews and vegetables.

SERVES 2

150g oyster mushrooms, broken into quarters

2 tbsp virgin olive oil

1/2 tsp garlic powder

1/2 tsp cumin powder

1/2 tsp smoked paprika

Good pinch of salt

Preheat oven to 170°C (350°F). Toss mushrooms in oil, spices and salt and spread on a flat tray lined with baking paper. Bake for 20–25 minutes or until mushrooms have crisped and browned.

celeriac remoulade & rare roast beef rolls

These are really easy to make and can be served as a starter or packed in a lunchbox. Rare roast beef can be purchased in most good delis. To make a homemade mayonnaise, see page 191.

MAKES 6 ROLLS

1/2 celeriac, peeled and sliced into matchstick-thin strips

1 tsp horseradish

1 tbsp mayonnaise

1 tbsp lemon juice

Pinch of pepper

2 tbsp chopped spring onion

1 tbsp chopped fresh parsley

6 slices of rare roast beef

Combine celeriac with everything but the beef. Place equal amounts of mix on the lower third of the beef slices and roll tightly upwards. Secure with a toothpick if needed.

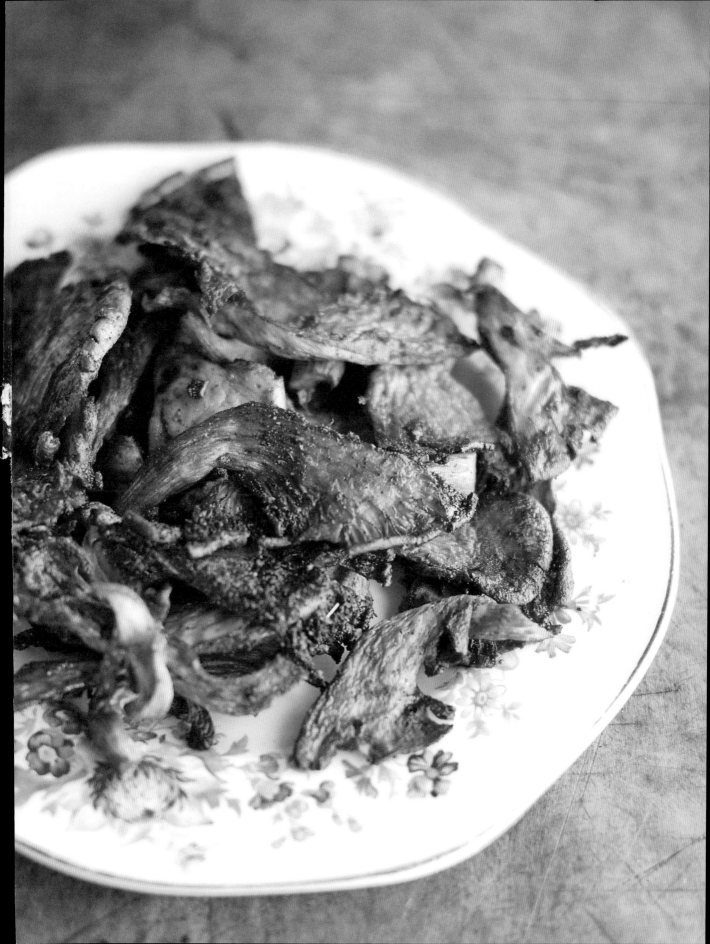

grilled haloumi with orange vanilla sauce

If you can tolerate a little dairy, especially the goat and sheep's milk kind, you will love the balance of salty, sweet and subtly sour flavours of this dish. Haloumi cheese is a regular in our fridge and this is a lovely way to serve it for a special dinner party.

SERVES 3-4 FOR APPETIZER

Juice of 2 oranges

Peel of 1 orange

Seeds from 1/2 vanilla pod, sliced lengthways

1 tbsp lemon juice

2/3 tsp of honey

Ghee or coconut oil for frying

250g haloumi cheese, sliced

A few orange slices, mint leaves and raw pistachio nuts to serve

Combine orange juice, orange peel, vanilla, lemon juice and honey in a saucepan and bring to simmer. Cook for 15 minutes or until thickened and syrupy. Remove candied orange peel and slice thinly.

Heat a little ghee or coconut oil to high. Slice and fry haloumi cheese for 1–2 minutes on each side, or until crispy and golden brown.

Assemble on a platter with fresh orange slices, pistachios, candied orange slices, mint and drizzled with orange syrup.

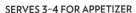
red chilli & kaffir lime almonds

MAKES 150G

150g raw almonds

1 tsp coconut oil

2/3 tsp dried red chilli flakes or chopped fresh red chilli

1 small garlic clove, finely chopped

1 tbsp finely chopped kaffir lime leaves (5 leaves)

Zest of 1 fresh lime

2 tbsp lime juice

1 tbsp tamari wheat-free soy sauce

1/2 tsp sea salt

Heat a large frying pan over medium–high heat. Add almonds and cook over medium heat for about 15 minutes, stirring very frequently to prevent burning, until lightly browned and smoky. Remove almonds to a side plate.

Add coconut oil, chilli, garlic, and kaffir lime leaves to the frying pan. Stir and cook on medium heat for about 30 seconds. Add back the almonds together with lime zest, lime juice, Tamari sauce and sea salt. Combine well and cook for another minute or two. Remove almonds to a wooden board or a large tray, ensuring all the seasoning is scraped off the frying pan and added to the almonds. Cool off completely before storing in an airtight container.

Keep for 2–3 days in an airtight container out of the fridge, or for up to a week in the refrigerator.

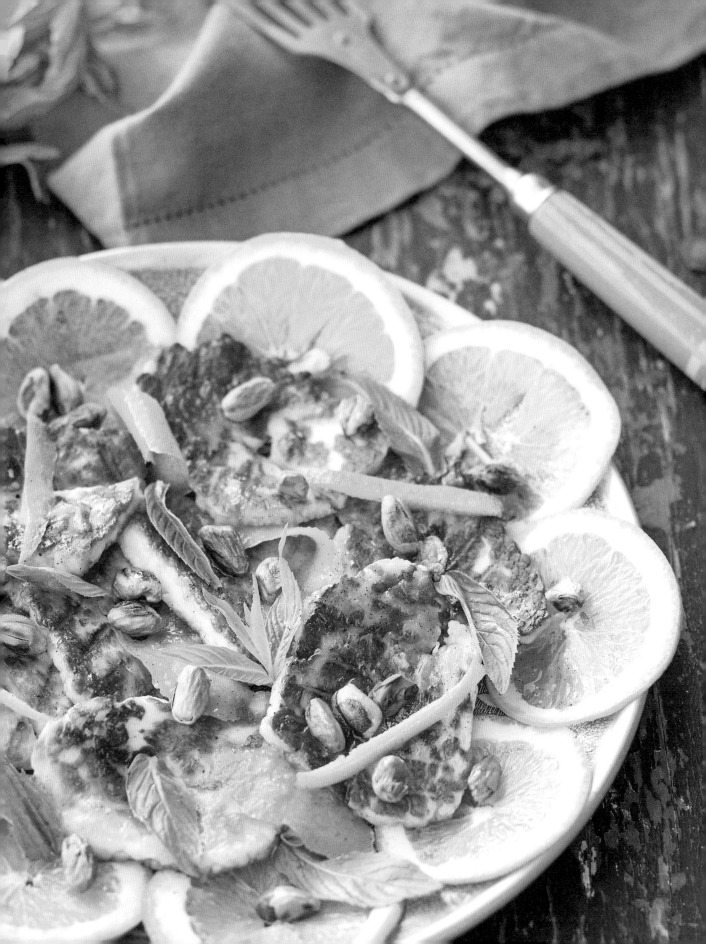

spicy sweet potato chips

Blink and they'll be gone, especially if you have kids hanging around. These are so much tastier than regular, deep-fried white potato chips. Plus, you'll be getting plenty of beta-carotene and vitamin C.

SERVES 4

2 medium sweet potatoes

4–5 tbsp virgin olive oil

2/3 tsp sea salt

1 tsp paprika

1 tsp cumin powder

1 tsp garlic powder

Pinch of red chilli flakes

Pinch of sea salt to serve

Preheat oven to 180°C (360°F).

Peel and cut sweet potatoes into chips, about 7mm wide. Toss in olive oil, salt and spices.

Place chips on two flat trays lined with baking paper, leaving a little space in between. Bake for 30 minutes or until a crispy and golden brown. I rotate the trays around to ensure even temperature and I turn some of the faster-cooking chips over halfway through. Sprinkle with a little more sea salt once ready and out of the oven.

spicy coconut prawns

SERVES 6

100g desiccated coconut

1 tsp onion powder

1 tsp garlic powder

1/2 tsp chilli powder or flakes

1/2 tsp Chinese five-spice powder

1 tsp sea salt

2 eggs

45g tapioca flour/starch

125ml coconut or macadamia oil

20 fresh green prawns, peeled leaving tails intact, deveined

Fresh lime wedges to serve

Mix coconut with onion, garlic and chilli powder, Chinese five-spice powder and salt in a bowl. In a separate bowl, whisk the eggs and place tapioca flour in a third bowl or a plate.

Heat oil in a deep frying pan or a wok. Dip each prawn into tapioca flour and shake off the excess. Then dip in the egg and the coconut mixture. Cook in oil, in batches, for 2 minutes on each side or until golden. Don't overcrowd the pan. Transfer cooked prawns to a plate lined with paper towel to soak up the excess oil. Serve with wedges of fresh lime or my South Eastern Express marinade (page 198) to dip in.

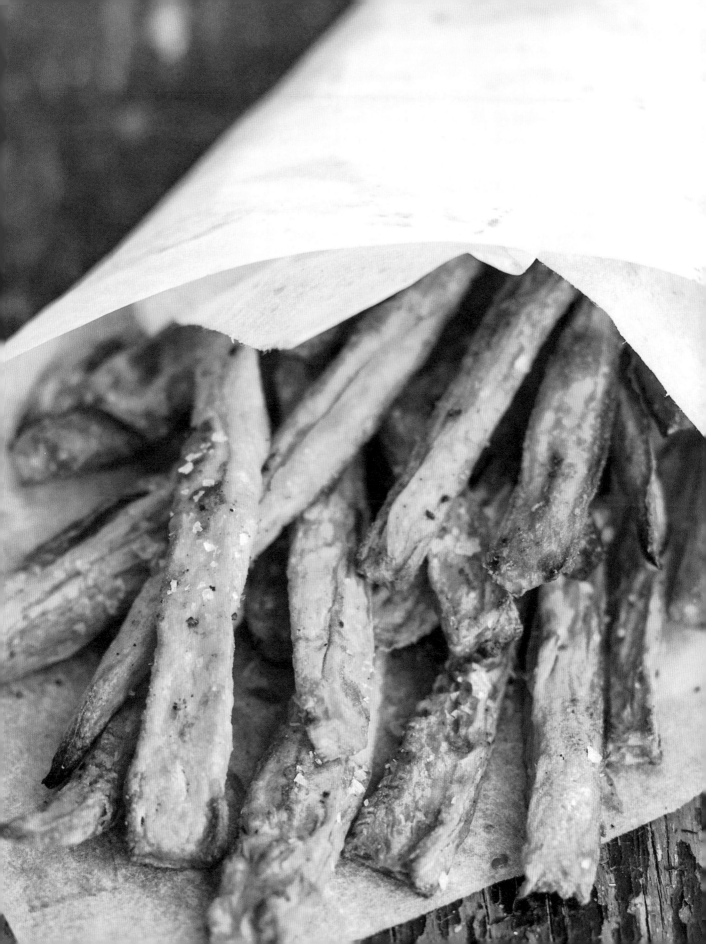

pickled onion tomato salad with pancetta

This vitamin-C-packed salad is a little beauty and you can make it as part of an antipasto platter or as a main side dish with grilled steak or fish. It reminds me of the food my grandmother used to make – lots of pickled vegetables, spices and strong flavours.

SERVES 3–4 AS PART OF A STARTER

1/2 tsp coriander seeds

1/4 tsp peppercorns

1 tsp mustard seeds

2 tbsp red wine vinegar

3/4 tsp sea salt

2 tbsp extra-virgin olive oil

1 large red onion, thinly sliced into whole rings

4 slices of pancetta

Ghee or coconut oil for cooking

About 18 small cherry tomatoes

Grind coriander seeds and peppercorns into powder using a mortar and pestle. Add to a bowl with mustard seeds, vinegar, salt and olive oil. Mix through the onion rings and set aside for at least 20 minutes before using. Pan-fry pancetta slices in a little ghee or coconut oil until crispy on both sides. Cut tomatoes in half and mix with pickled onion and pieces of crispy pancetta.

You can use pre-ground coriander seed and pepper instead. Prosciutto and even bacon can be used instead of pancetta.

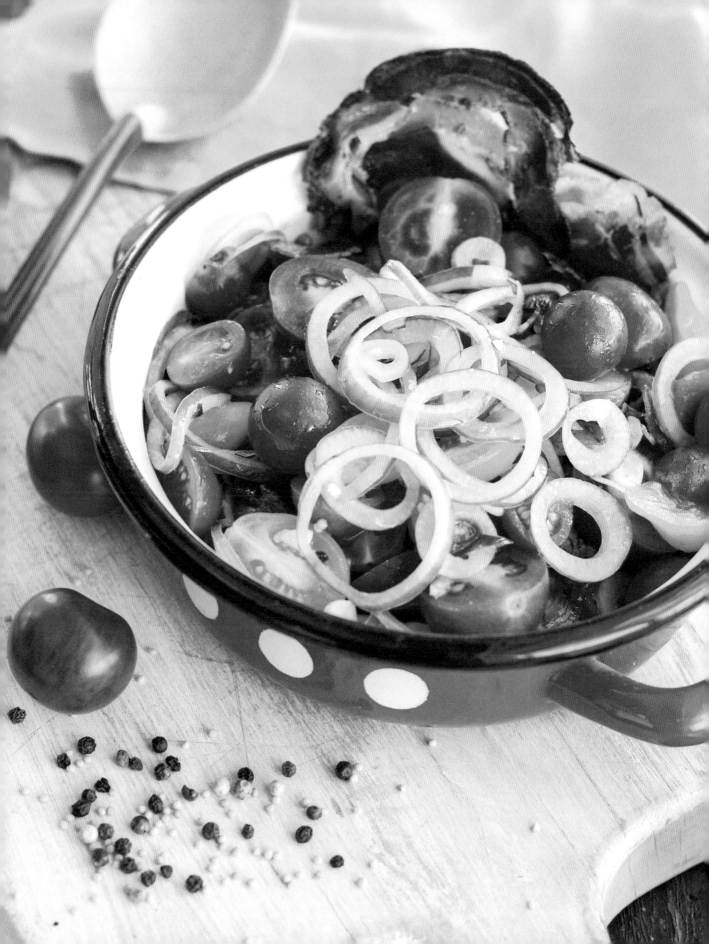

tahini & wholegrain crackers

MAKES 12-15 CRACKERS

3 tbsp tahini paste

1 tbsp soft butter, ghee or coconut oil

1 egg

2 tbsp sesame seeds

Pinch of salt

1 tbsp wholegrain mustard

2 1/2 tbsp coconut flour

Preheat oven to 170°C (338°F).

Mix tahini, butter, egg, sesame seeds, salt and mustard in a bowl until well combined. Add coconut flour and mix until thick, sticky mixture forms. Coconut flour absorbs lots of moisture and is therefore used sparingly, which means you will need to increase the amount if using different flour.

Roll the mixture into a ball and place on a slightly greased parchment/baking paper (about 40cm x 40cm). Using your hands, flatten the dough into a flat pancake. Then cover with another piece of parchment paper of the same size and use a rolling pin to flatten the pancake into a thin dough layer, about 3–5mm. Roll evenly in four directions starting from the middle. Remove the top piece of paper and use a knife to make small incision marks vertically and horizontally to make it easier to break the crackers when cooked.

Leaving the dough on the parchment paper, place it on the middle oven shelf and cook for about 12–15 minutes. When the outer edges start going golden brown, remove the tray from the oven and detach the outer crackers. Place the tray back in the oven for a further 4–5 minutes.

Remove the remaining part from the oven when lightly golden brown, leave to cool and separate into individual crackers. Keep in an airtight container for up to 5–6 days.

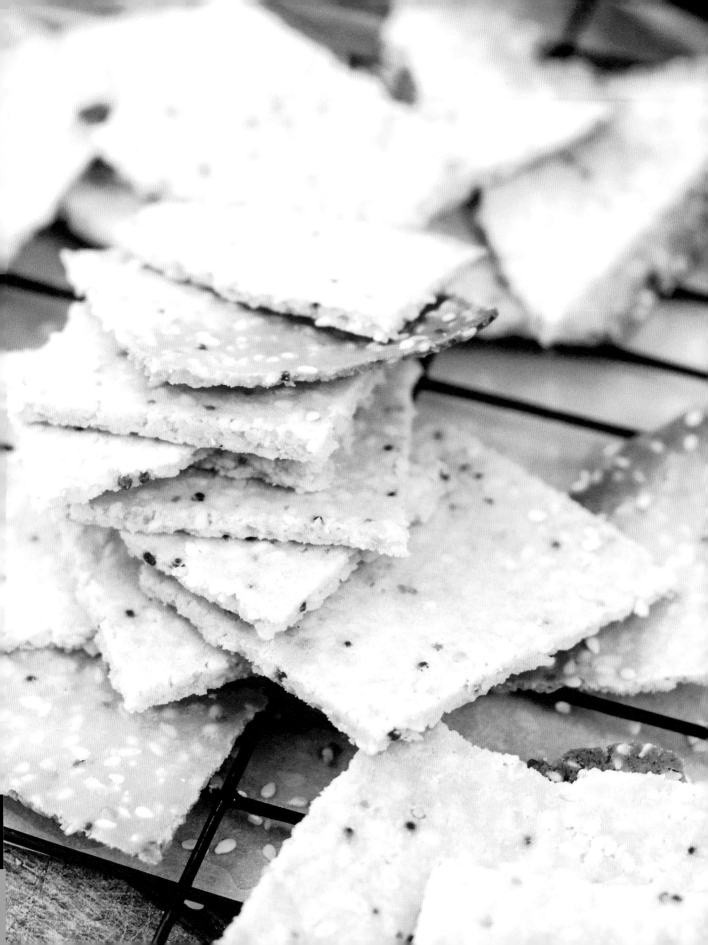

asian prawn & pork rolls

MAKES 12 ROLLS

1 tbsp coconut oil

3 shallots, finely chopped

1 tsp grated ginger

1/2 long red chilli, chopped

200g pork mince

4–5 shitake mushrooms (fresh or dried), chopped

1 garlic clove, finely chopped

1 tbsp fish sauce

2 tsp coconut aminos

1 tbsp lime juice

12 cooked king prawns, peeled

1 Chinese cabbage, leaves separated

Handful of fresh coriander leaves

Handful of fresh mint leaves

1 large carrot, peeled and grated

Heat coconut oil in a wok or a frying pan and fry shallots, ginger and chilli until softened. Add pork and shitake mushrooms and cook until slightly browned. Add garlic, fish sauce, coconut aminos and lime juice and cook together for a further 6–7 minutes until pork is well cooked. Remove to a plate.

Meanwhile, peel and cut the prawns in halves and boil some water in a large saucepan. Wash the cabbage leaves and blanch in boiling water for about 40–50 seconds. You can drop them in the water in batches. Remove and rinse under cold water to stop the cooking process. Pat dry with a tea towel and trim off the thicker part of the leaf at the bottom.

Place a tablespoon of pork filling in the centre of each leaf. Top with a couple of prawn halves, a few coriander and mint leaves and a little grated carrot. Fold both sides on the bottom inwards and roll up into a tight roll. Serve with my Asian Twang dressing (page 196) as a dipping sauce.

If using dry shitake mushrooms, soak them in some warm water for 10 minutes to rehydrate before frying. You can use a little palm sugar and gluten-free soy sauce instead of coconut aminos. Normal white cabbage leaves can also be used; however, they should be blanched for a just a little bit longer. You could also use fresh cos lettuce and make smaller rolls. Omit chilli if avoiding nightshades.

Make
YOUR
OWN

cashew hummus

MAKES 250ML

190g cashews

2 tbsp lemon juice

2 tbsp tahini paste

2 tbsp extra-virgin olive oil

1 garlic clove

125ml water

2/3 tsp sea salt + pinch of pepper

Soak cashews in warm water and a teaspoon of lemon juice or white wine vinegar for 5–6 hours. Rinse well and transfer to a food processor. Add the rest of ingredients and process for 3–4 minutes, scraping the sides as you go, until very smooth and thick. Add extra water to get a thinner consistency or to dilute the flavour if you find lemon or garlic overpowering. Keep refrigerated for up to a week. Blanched almonds or cauliflower can be used instead of cashews.

lemony harissa

This recipe is a result of multiple experimentations and adaptations of different harissa sauces. It's rich and spicy, and when drizzled over grilled lamb – it's a match made in heaven.

MAKES ABOUT 250ML

1 tsp whole fennel seeds

2 tsp coriander seeds

2 tsp cumin seeds

2 tsp tomato purée

125ml extra-virgin olive oil

Zest and juice of 1/2 lemon

1/4 preserved lemon, chopped

1/2 tsp caraway seeds

1/2 tsp smoked paprika

1/2 tsp sea salt

2/3 tsp coconut syrup or honey

1 tbsp chopped fresh coriander

1 long red chilli, chopped

60ml water

Using a mortar and pestle or a food processor, grind fennel, coriander and cumin seeds into rough powder. Transfer to a food processor and add the rest of ingredients. Process into smooth paste, taste and add more chilli for extra heat if preferred. Keep refrigerated in a glass container for one to two weeks.

Lemony harissa can be used to marinate lamb, beef or chicken or used on top of grilled seafood. It can also be added to Middle East-inspired stews and African tagines. Preserved lemons can be purchased from most supermarkets and delis, or made at home.

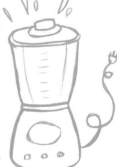

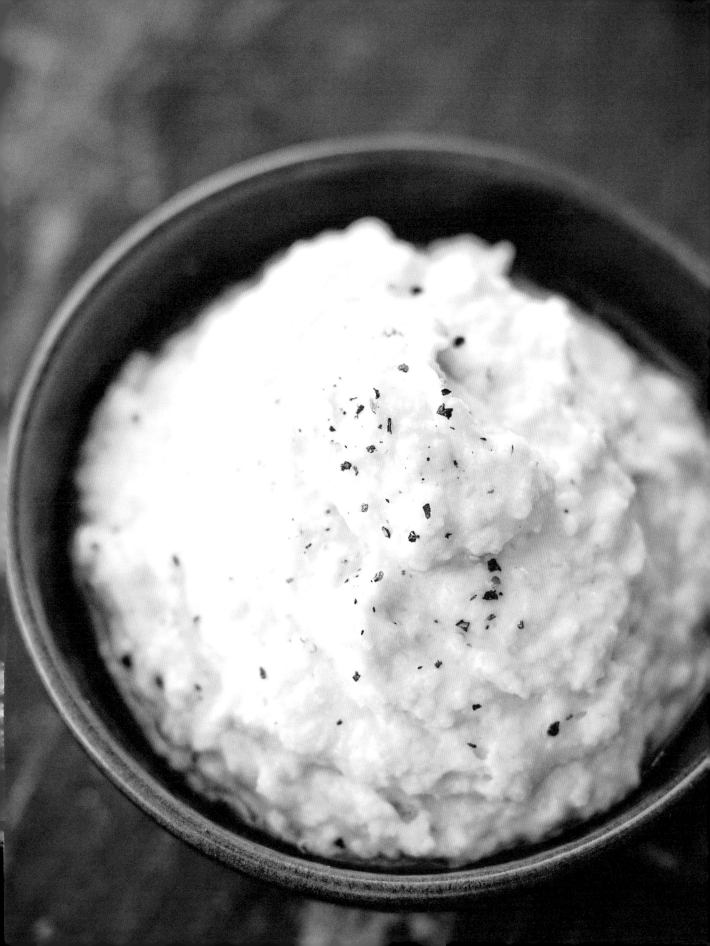

roasted tomato ketchupy sauce

I've been looking for a good recipe for tomato sauce/tomato ketchup that didn't use added sugar and wasn't flavoured with enhancers or other nasty additives. After a few experiments, this is what I came up with. It's inspired by a few different methods and my own little twists. I used carrots and roasted tomatoes, both of which caramelise and provide sweetness during cooking.

MAKES TWO BOTTLES

500g fresh ripe roma or plum tomatoes, cut into quarters

Virgin olive oil

1 tsp salt

1 medium brown onion, peeled and finely diced

1 stick celery, finely diced

2 medium carrots, peeled and finely grated

Thumb-sized nub of fresh ginger, finely grated

2 garlic cloves, peeled and chopped

1/2 fresh red chilli (or a pinch of chilli flakes)

1 tsp smoked paprika

1 tsp good quality fish sauce

1 tbsp dried or fresh oregano leaves

1 tbsp coriander seeds

3 cloves

2 bay leaves

Pinch of sea salt

1 tsp ground black pepper

375ml organic canned tomatoes, chopped

125ml red wine vinegar

250ml water

Preheat oven to 170°C (350°F). Toss fresh tomatoes in some olive oil and salt and spread on a foil-covered tray. Roast in the oven for 30 minutes.

Place onion, celery and carrots in a heavy-bottom medium saucepan with a few tablespoons of olive oil. Cook over a low heat for 15 minutes until softened, stirring occasionally.

Add ginger, garlic, chilli, paprika, fish sauce, oregano, coriander seeds, cloves, bay leaves, salt and pepper. Cook for a minute and add roasted tomatoes, canned tomatoes, vinegar and water. Bring to boil and simmer gently until the sauce reduces in half.

Transfer to a food processor and purée until well blended. Push the sauce through a sieve to discard any skin or unblended ingredients. Place the sauce back on the heat and simmer for a further 15 minutes to thicken. Check seasoning and add more salt or vinegar. Pour the ketchup into sterilised jars or bottles, seal tightly and keep in the fridge for up to three months.

bone broth

I remember my grandmother had a huuuge pot in which she often boiled a bunch of bones. She would use the gelatine-rich liquid to make 'holodetz', a traditional dish of soft-cooked meat covered in meat stock jelly. I loved the taste but I had no idea how nutritious that dish was. Today, homemade bone broth is going through a bit of a renaissance. Forget about 'an apple a day keeps the doctor away', it's all about having a daily cup of homemade bone broth to heal your gut, improve immunity, reduce joint and arthritis pain and to keep our nails, skin and hair looking healthy and beautiful.

MAKES 3 1/2 LITRES

2.5kg mixed bones (beef marrow, knuckle bone and some meatier bones like ribs and neck)

3 tbsp white wine vinegar

3–4 litres of cold water

2 brown onions, cut into quarters

2 large carrots, roughly cut

2 celery stalks, roughly cut

1 tsp black or mixed colour peppercorns

1 tbsp salt

3 garlic cloves

1 star anise

Bouquet garni (thyme, bay leaf and parsley tied together with a string)

Bone broth can be drunk like a soup, used as a stock base for casseroles and stews, used to braise vegetables and to make sauces and gravy.

Place the bones with less meat in a pot with vinegar and cover with water. The acidity of the vinegar will help release the nutrients from the bones. Set aside for 30–40 minutes. In the meantime, place the meatier bones in a roasting tray and cook in the oven, at 170°C (350°F), for 40 minutes or until browned.

Add roasted bones to the stockpot and bring everything to boil. Some of the impurities will float to the top as grayish foam. Skim it off with a slotted spoon.

Add vegetables (not including garlic or herbs), peppercorns and salt. Bring back to boil and then turn the heat down to gentle simmer. Cook for about 12 hours. Check every 20 minutes for the first hour or two to remove any new scum that floats to the top. Add garlic, star anise and bouquet garni in the last two hours of cooking.

Once the cooking time is up, remove the bones with tongs or a slotted spoon. Strain the stock into a large container or a bowl (it won't look pretty at this point). Cool the liquid in the fridge and then remove the congealed fat that forms at the top with a spoon. Transfer the stock to smaller containers and keep some in the fridge for immediate use and some in the freezer for longer-term storage.

red chilli dip

This lovely dip is full of big flavours. Eat with your favourite crispy vegetables or use as a stuffing for mushrooms and meatballs.

MAKES 375ML

100g soaked cashews

1 tsp lemon juice (or white vinegar)

10 sundried tomatoes, sliced

1 tbsp tomato purée

1/2 large red pepper, chopped

1 garlic clove, chopped

2 tbsp red wine vinegar

125ml extra-virgin olive oil

1 long red chilli, chopped

2 pinches of salt

Pinch of pepper

A splash of water

Soak cashews in warm water and a teaspoon of lemon juice or white wine vinegar for 5–6 hours. Rinse well and transfer to a food processor. Add the rest of ingredients and process for 3–4 minutes, scraping the sides as you go, until very smooth and thick.

Keep refrigerated for up to a week.

creamy spinach & egg dip

MAKES 375ML

1 bunch of fresh spinach

5 hard-boiled eggs, peeled

1 garlic clove, peeled and grated

2 tbsp finally chopped spring onion

3 tbsp mayonnaise

1/2 tsp sea salt and pepper

1 tbsp lemon juice

Bring a saucepan of water to boil or use the water after boiling the eggs. Cook spinach in boiling water for about 30 seconds. Rinse under cold water, squeeze the moisture out and chop roughly. Place the spinach with the rest of ingredients in a food processor and purée until smooth and well combined. Alternatively, chop everything finely and combine in a bowl.

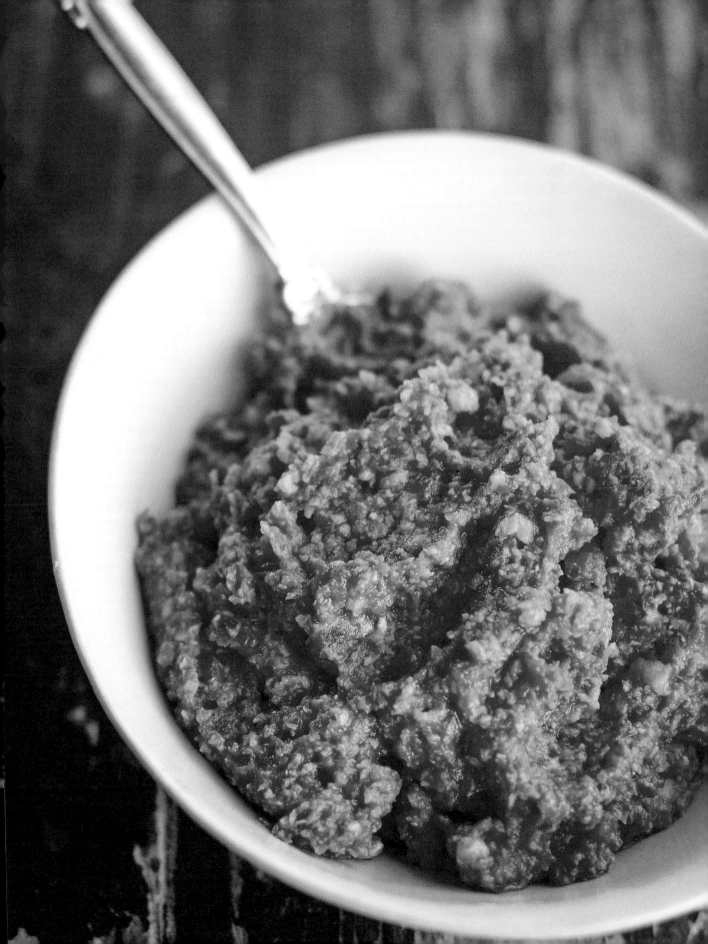

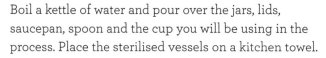

homemade coconut yoghurt

There is only one thing you need to know about making your own coconut yoghurt – it's a lot easier than you think. Once you get the tools and the ingredients, there is really not that much to it. It tastes just like any other natural yoghurt but with a light coconut flavour. Perfect for keeping your gut flora healthy and your morning granola as tasty as ever.

MAKES ABOUT 750ML

For the yoghurt

2 cans of coconut cream (400ml each)

3/4 tsp yoghurt culture/starter

Equipment

A thermometer

2 clean jars with lids

A cooler bag

A kitchen towel

A saucepan

A small cup and a spoon

> You can purchase a yoghurt starter culture in powder form from most health food stores, usually found in the refrigerated section. You can use some of the previous yoghurt as a culture for your new yoghurt.

Boil a kettle of water and pour over the jars, lids, saucepan, spoon and the cup you will be using in the process. Place the sterilised vessels on a kitchen towel.

Pour coconut cream into a medium saucepan, reserving as much of the watery liquid that sinks to the bottom as possible. Gently heat to 43°C (110°F); use a thermometer by placing it halfway into the liquid. Remove from heat.

Add 1 tablespoon of warm coconut cream to a clean cup. Add the culture powder and stir until it forms a paste. Add a little more liquid and stir again. Pour the mix back into the main saucepan and stir.

Pour coconut cream mix into glass jars and seal with a lid. Wrap jars in a kitchen towel and place in the cooler bag. Essentially we want to maintain the temperature close to 40°C for as long as possible and that's why you need something with insulation (alternatively, you could wrap the jars in foil and some towels). Leave in a warm place for 12 hours. Then take jars out of the bag and place in the fridge for another 12 hours before eating.

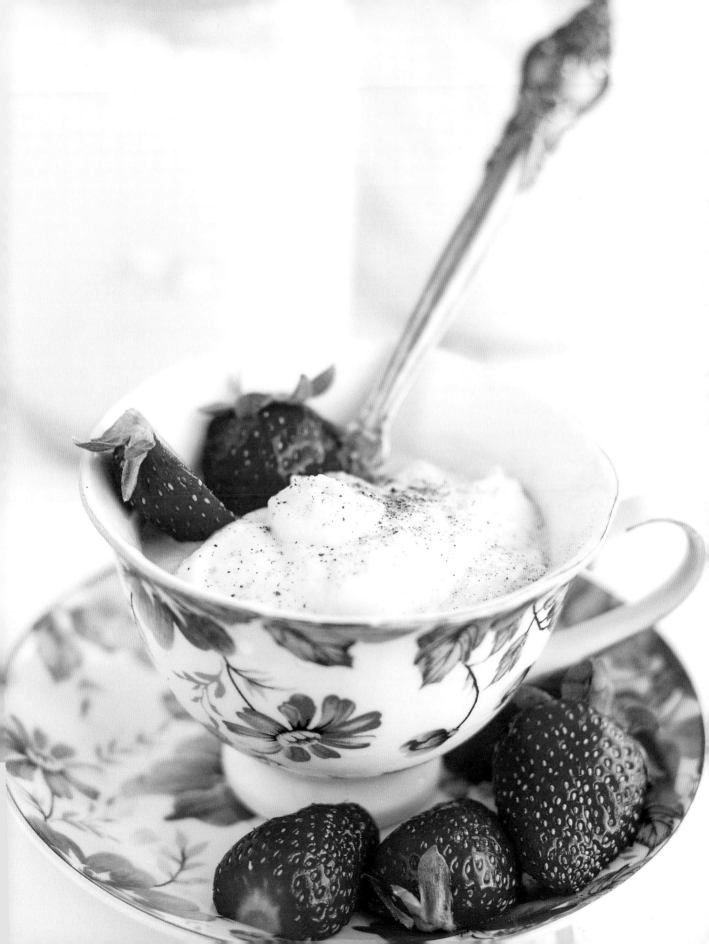

garlic jam

MAKES 375ML

About 30 unpeeled garlic cloves

1 medium brown onion, sliced

10 sundried tomatoes, sliced

3 tbsp macadamia oil (or ghee)

4 tbsp coconut syrup or raw honey

Zest and juice from 1 lemon

2 tsp salt

1/2 tsp ground black pepper

1/2 tsp coriander seed powder

250ml vegetable stock

1 tsp red chilli flakes

You can do a similar jam with roasted onions or leeks. The jam can be used as a condiment with grilled meats and fish, eggs or stirred through casseroles and sauces to add some of that beautiful sweet yet subtle garlic flavour.

Preheat oven to 170°C (350°F). Spread garlic cloves in a large roasting tray and spray with olive oil. Bake in the oven for 30 minutes.

Meanwhile, sauté onion and sundried tomatoes in macadamia oil or ghee in a medium saucepan for about 7 minutes, until onion is softened.

Once garlic is cooked, remove from the oven and set aside until cooled down enough to touch. Cut the root ends off and peel the cloves, trying to keep them intact. Add peeled garlic cloves to onion and tomatoes together with coconut syrup or honey, lemon juice, lemon zest, salt, pepper, coriander, vegetable stock and chilli flakes. Bring to boil, then turn to simmer and cook on low heat for 1 hour, stirring through a few times. The mixture will thicken and caramelise.

Let it cool down to room temperature before transferring to sterilised jars. Cover the top with a piece of plastic wrap and an airtight lid. Keep in the fridge for up to two months.

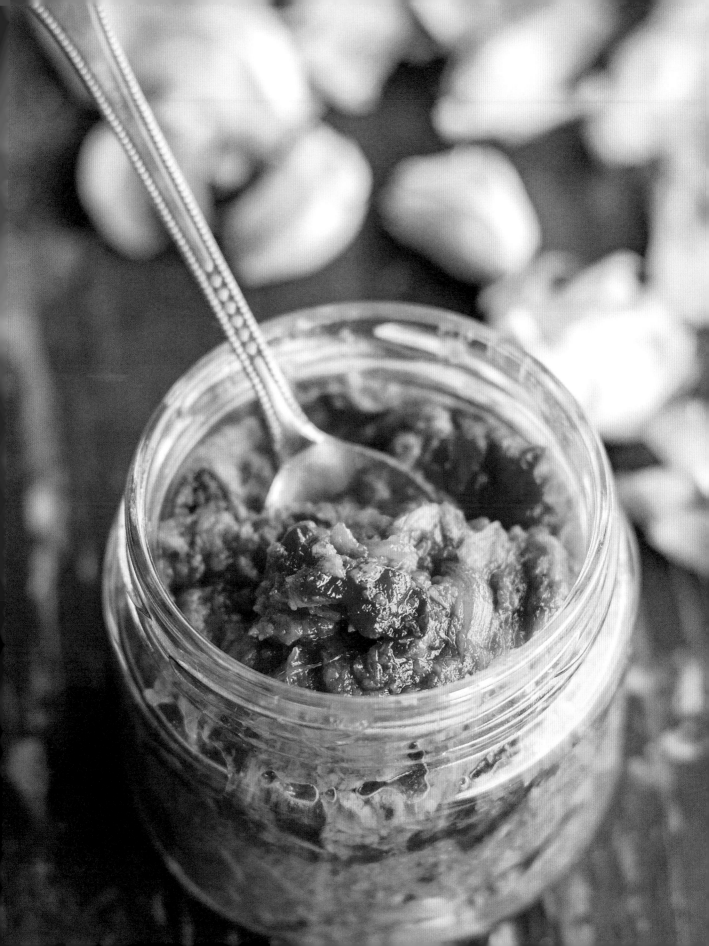

beef jerky

Beef jerky is a popular snack but it can be a little expensive, and you can't always find a brand that uses natural ingredients. Make sure the beef is grass fed and lean, as fatty cuts can go rancid with storage.

MAKES 300G

500g beef fillet, washed and pat-dried

1 tsp smoked paprika

2 tsp coriander seed powder

1 tsp garlic powder

1 tsp onion powder

2 1/2 tsp sea salt

1 tsp ground black pepper

1 tsp red chilli flakes

Place beef fillets in the freezer for 30 minutes or for long enough to firm up but not harden completely. This will make it easier to slice it into thin strips.

Mix spices and coat beef fillet strips. Cover and leave in the fridge for 12 hours.

Preheat oven to 70°C (160°F). Remove a rack from the oven and make sure it's clean. Lay meat strips directly on the oven rack so that air can circulate around them. Line the bottom of the oven with some foil to catch the drippings. Place the rack in the oven and cook the strips for 3 hours, turning them over halfway through. Then partially open the oven letting the temperature go down to around 45°C (110°F). Dehydrate with the door partially open for another 3–4 hours, or until the jerky is darkened and cracks when bent. Remove the rack and let the jerky cool down completely before storing.

Go for lean cuts of beef. Homemade jerky can be stored in a pantry for a few days but ideally should be stored in the fridge wrapped in plastic or in an airtight container. It will last for a good month.

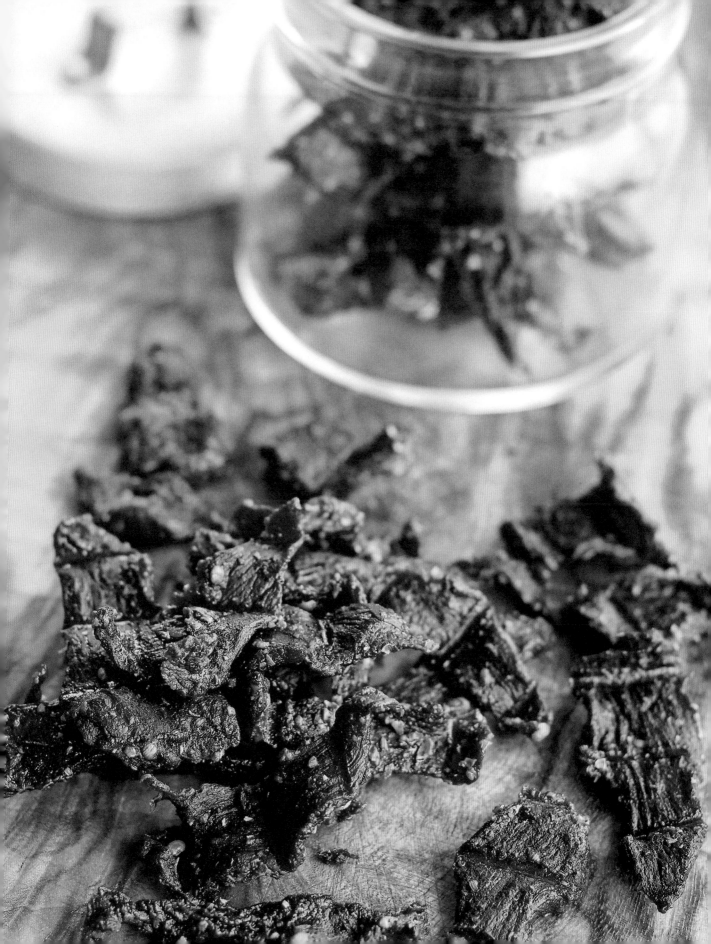

purple sauerkraut

Sauerkraut is somewhat of a staple in Ukrainian cuisine and I often watched my parents make large batches of fermented cabbage in none other than a bathtub. Yep, that's how much sour cabbage we went through, especially in winter when many fresh vegetables were out of season. Fresh sauerkraut is a fantastic addition to your meals as the fermentation process develops probiotics, essential for healthy gut. Start with a small batch using this recipe before you attempt a bathtub amount.

MAKES 250–375ML

1/4 large purple cabbage head (or half a smaller head)

1 medium carrot, grated

1 garlic clove

1/2 tsp coriander seed powder

1 1/2 tbsp sea salt

Water

Other common spices and flavours to add to your sauerkraut are caraway seeds, dill seeds, mustard seeds, celery seeds, juniper berries, onion, chilli, turmeric and ginger. You can use some of the leftover fresh sauerkraut to mix in with a new batch of salted cabbage to kick-start the fermentation process.

Thinly slice or shred the cabbage, discarding the core. Using your hands, squeeze and mix cabbage, carrot, garlic, coriander and sea salt in a large mixing bowl. Use a meat hammer or a wooden spoon to pound the mix for a few minutes to release the juices. Alternatively – and this is what I do – you can place a saucer or a small plate on top of the mixture inside the bowl, cover it with plastic wrap, put a small kettle bell on top of the plate and press it down gently. Leave it for a couple of hours to release more liquid.

Meanwhile, sterilise a medium glass jar with some boiling water and let it dry. Place the cabbage mix tightly in the jar, pressing it down with a spoon or your clean hand to release more juice to the top. Leave a 2cm space between the top of the jar and the cabbage. Make sure the cabbage is completely covered with brine. Cover tightly and leave at room temperature for about 3 days before moving to the fridge. The vegetables will soften and change colour slightly and when you open the lid, it should smell acidic and sharp. If any mould forms on the top, gently remove it. The sauerkraut can be eaten straight away or left in the fridge for months.

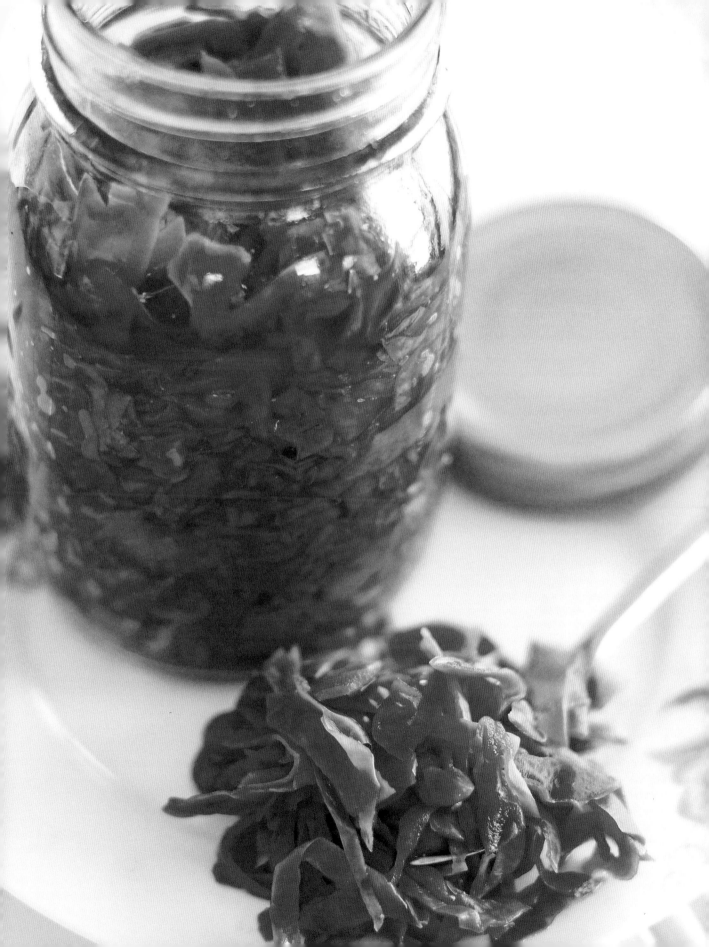

cashew satay sauce

Use satay sauce to serve with chicken, beef or lamb skewers, or to make into a slightly thinner sauce for Indonesian Gado Gado salad with lots of cooked and raw vegetables, boiled eggs and fresh herbs. Visit Eat Drink Paleo website for more pictures.

MAKES 250ML

3 small red chillies, deseeded

2 garlic cloves, roughly chopped

1 lemongrass stalk, two outer layers removed and roughly chopped

3 small shallots, peeled and roughly chopped

2 tsp curry powder

1 tsp turmeric powder

1 1/2 tbsp coconut oil

400g unsalted raw cashews

375ml water

150ml coconut milk

Juice of 1/2 lime

2 tbsp coconut aminos (or naturally brewed, gluten-free soy sauce)

3 tsp fish sauce

1 tbsp honey

Pinch of sea salt

Process chillies, garlic, lemongrass, shallots, and curry and turmeric powders to a smooth paste or use a mortar and pestle to grind ingredients together.

Heat coconut oil in a small saucepan. Add the ground paste and fry for about 4–5 minutes on medium heat, stirring frequently to prevent sticking. The mixture will start caramelising and browning slightly.

Meanwhile, heat a large frying pan on medium heat and toast cashew nuts for 2 minutes, stirring frequently to prevent burning. You will be stirring the nuts and the mixture in parallel.

Add 250ml of water to the paste and bring to boil. Grind toasted cashews into crumbs using a food processor. Add to the cooking mixture together with coconut milk, lime juice, coconut aminos and fish sauce. Bring to boil and then bring the heat down to simmer. Cook for 5 minutes and add honey, a good pinch of salt (about 2/3 teaspoon) and the rest of the of water. Cook for a further 4–5 minutes, stirring frequently as the mixture will start thickening and caramelising. Take off the heat and transfer to a blender to further process into a smooth paste, adding a little more water if needed.

Store in the fridge in a sterilised airtight jar. To sterilise the jar, give it a good wash, then rinse the lid and the jar with boiling water.

homemade mayo

When I transitioned into paleo I had a mini panic attack because I thought mayonnaise would be a complete no-no. For me, it's been its own food group for most of my life. Thankfully, it's very much paleo friendly as it is essentially an egg yolk and oil emulsion with some mustard, vinegar and salt. This recipe is an adaptation from US chef Julia Child's method.

Make sure all ingredients are at room temperature. Warm a large bowl in hot water and dry it. Add the egg yolks and beat for 1–2 minutes until thick and sticky. Add the vinegar or lemon juice, salt and mustard. Beat for 30 seconds more. The egg yolks are now ready to receive the oil.

Add oil drop by drop at the start. Keep beating constantly until the sauce has thickened. Add the drops of oil with a teaspoon, or rest the lip of the bottle on the edge of the bowl. Keep your eye on the oil rather than on the sauce. Stop pouring every 10 seconds or so but continue beating to be sure the egg yolks are absorbing the oil.

After 80–125ml of oil has been incorporated, the sauce will thicken into a heavy cream and the potential crisis of curdling is over. Beat in the remaining oil by amounts of 1–2 tablespoons, blending it thoroughly after each addition. When the sauce becomes too thick and stiff, beat in drops of vinegar or lemon juice to thin it out. Then continue with the oil.

Finally, beat the boiling water into the sauce. This is an anti-curdling insurance. Season to taste. If the sauce is not used immediately, scrape it into a small bowl and cover it tightly to prevent a skin forming on its surface.

MAKES 500ML

3 egg yolks

1 tablespoon wine vinegar or lemon juice (more drops as needed to taste)

2/3 teaspoon salt

1/2 teaspoon dry or prepared mustard

375ml of macadamia oil (at room temperature)

2 tablespoons boiling water

The maximum amount of oil one egg yolk can absorb is about 180ml, after which the binding properties of the egg break down and the sauce starts to thin and curdle. The safest amount is 125ml of oil per egg yolk. The proportions of ingredients look something like this:
2 egg yolks + 250ml fat (oil) + 2–3 tablespoons vinegar/ lemon juice = about 375ml mayonnaise.

red curry paste

Having some red curry paste on hand is very useful as you can toss it in a stir-fry or mix it with some coconut milk for a quick pumpkin or chicken curry. It's also great for marinating meats and seafood. You might have to make a trip to an Asian store or fresh food market for some of the ingredients.

MAKES 250ML

3 shallots, chopped

4 garlic cloves, roughly chopped

2 long red chillies, chopped with seeds

1 lemongrass stalk, sliced

1 1/2 tbsp grated galangal, peel first

1 1/2 tbsp grated turmeric, peel first

7 kaffir lime leaves

3 fresh coriander stalks, chopped

1 1/2 tbsp fish sauce

2 tbsp virgin olive oil

1/2 tsp grated palm sugar

1/2 tsp shrimp paste (optional)

To make the curry paste, place all ingredients in a food processor and purée into as smooth a paste as possible, for about 2–3 minutes. Keep in the fridge, in an airtight container, covered with a layer of olive oil for up to seven days.

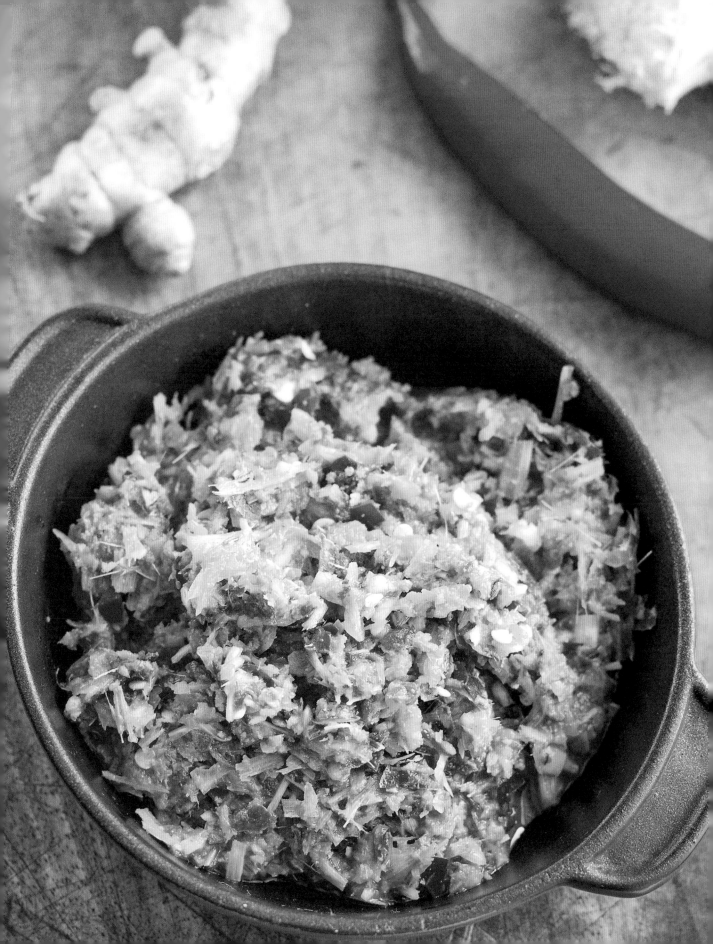

three butters

I love butter – for its lush texture, its ability to make everything taste better and its amazing nutritional profile. Even those avoiding dairy can indulge in a little butter given that it's mostly fat with very few milk solids left. These three butters are very versatile in the kitchen and can be kept in a fridge or a freezer, ready to smother grilled fish, steak or a stack of pancakes.

Place all ingredients in a food processor and purée until well combined. Refrigerate in a glass or safe plastic container.

LIME & CORIANDER BUTTER

100g soft butter

2 tbsp chopped fresh coriander

Zest and juice of 1 lime

1/2 tsp sea salt

1/2 tsp ground black pepper

Use on grilled fish, prawns, scallops or chicken; toss with spinach, broccoli or green peas, or melt over savoury muffins and fritters.

STRAWBERRY BUTTER

100g soft butter

10 fresh strawberries, finely chopped

1 tsp vanilla extract

Eat by the spoonful, melt over muffins and pancakes, or mix with some puréed cashews or macadamia nuts as a frosting for cupcakes.

SIMPLE CAFÉ DE PARIS BUTTER

100g soft butter

1 tsp Dijon mustard

2 anchovies, chopped

1 tbsp gluten-free Worcestershire sauce

1 tbsp capers, drained

1/2 tsp sea salt

1/2 tsp black pepper

1 garlic clove, diced

2 sprigs fresh thyme, leaves only

1/2 tsp curry powder

1 tsp lemon juice

Amazing on grilled red meat, roasts, baked sweet potatoes, roasted asparagus and mushrooms; for flavouring meatballs, and for finishing off meat casseroles, sauces and stews.

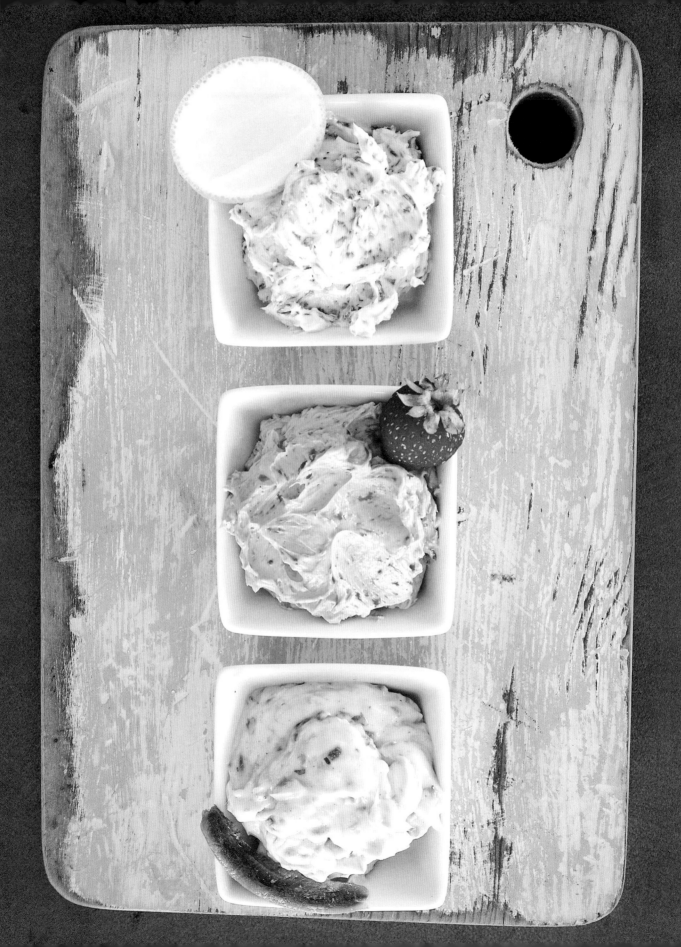

beloved salad dressings

These dressings are more like idea starters: I wanted to give you something fun, exotic, maybe a little weird even. Rest assured they are all delicious and you can enjoy them over cold and warm salads, vegetables, meats and seafood. For all dressings except the avocado ranch and tomato zing, whisk all ingredients in a bowl.

ASIAN TWANG

MAKES 80ML

1 tsp sesame oil

2 tbsp extra-virgin olive oil

1/2 small red chilli, chopped

1 small nub of fresh ginger, chopped

1 tbsp fish sauce

1 1/2 tbsp fresh lime juice

1/2 tsp grated palm sugar

1 tbsp freshly chopped coriander

Use for Asian coleslaw, Thai beef salad, oysters or over a grilled piece of fish. Toss through some Asian greens or use as a dipping sauce for grilled chicken wings.

HAZELNUT & VANILLA

MAKES 80ML

1 tsp vanilla extract

1 tbsp hazelnut oil

2 tbsp extra-virgin olive oil

35g hazelnuts, roasted and roughly chopped

1/2 tsp honey

1/2 tsp Dijon mustard

1 tbsp apple cider vinegar

1/4 tsp garlic powder

Drizzle over roasted pumpkin and carrots, or it's absolutely amazing over grilled aubergine. Also perfect over some rocket and beetroot with grilled lamb. Oh, and grilled calamari and prawns.

TAHINI & GARLIC

MAKES 160ML

Zest and juice of 1 lemon

1 tbsp tahini

1 garlic clove, finely grated

125ml extra-virgin olive oil

1/2 tsp cumin seed powder

Pinch of sea salt and black pepper

Really good with a beetroot and goat's cheese salad, pear salad, green bean salad or over roasted leeks. You could also try an autumn salad of roasted sweet potato, red onion and hazelnuts.

TOMATO ZING

MAKES 250ML

Juice of 2 lemons

1 garlic clove

30g sundried tomatoes

160ml extra-virgin olive oil

1/2 tsp sea salt

1/2 tsp chilli flakes or chopped chilli

1 tsp Dijon mustard

1 tsp lemon zest

Process all ingredients in a blender or a food processor until smooth.

beloved salad dressings

If making in larger batches, store in clean, air-tight glass jars in the fridge for up to one week.

TUTTI FRUTTI

MAKES 160ML

1/2 tsp grated lemon zest

1/2 tsp grated lime zest

1/2 tsp grated orange zest

2 tbsp orange juice

1 tbsp lime juice

1 tbsp lemon juice

1 tsp onion powder

1 tsp Dijon mustard

1 tbsp chopped fresh basil

125ml extra-virgin olive oil

2/3 tsp sea salt

1/2 tsp ground black pepper

This dressing is great on top of a ceviche or freshly grilled tuna or salmon; and in crispy summer salads with radishes, fennel, rocket, spinach, cherry tomatoes or cucumbers.

AVOCADO RANCH

MAKES 160ML

1 ripe avocado, mashed

1 tbsp coconut cream

1 tbsp white wine vinegar

1 tbsp extra-virgin olive oil

60ml water

1 tsp Dijon mustard

2 tbsp mixed chopped chives, parsley and dill (dried herbs can also be used)

1/2 tsp onion powder

1/2 tsp garlic powder

2/3 tsp sea salt

1/2 tsp white pepper

Use this thicker consistency dressing for burgers, coleslaw, sweet potato fries, Mexican pulled pork, paleo pizza sauce, or for dipping grilled prawns, chicken bites or vegetable crudités.

Process all ingredients in a blender or a food processor until smooth.

top-notch marinades

Marinating meat and seafood before cooking infuses flavour and kicks off the cooking process by softening the main ingredient. Below are calculated for about 500g of meat. Use a food processor to purée or whisk in a bowl.

BRONTE BEACH SUMMERS

125ml virgin olive oil

2 tbsp balsamic vinegar

2 tbsp gluten-free Worcestershire sauce

1 tsp garlic, finely diced

1 tsp sweet paprika

1 tsp sea salt

1/2 tsp ground black pepper

1 tsp dried Italian herbs or fresh parsley

Great with red meat, especially beef and lamb.

ARABIC NIGHTS

1 tsp ground cumin seeds

1 tsp ground coriander seeds

1 tsp ground caraway seeds

1 tsp turmeric powder

1 quarter preserved lemon, finely chopped

1 tbsp lemon juice

1 tsp tahini

1 tsp sea salt

125ml virgin olive oil

Rub all over lamb, goat, beef or chicken. It's great with vegetables too: try it on aubergines, carrots, pumpkin and red peppers. Add a spoonful to stews and tagines for a flavour kick.

SOUTH EASTERN EXPRESS

1 tbsp fish sauce

1 tbsp honey

1 tbsp naturally brewed, gluten-free soy sauce

1 tsp grated fresh garlic

1 tsp grated fresh ginger

1/2 tsp chilli flakes

1 tbsp lime juice

1 tsp sesame oil

2 tbsp virgin olive oil

Make tantalising chicken wings and drumsticks, beef skewers, grilled prawns or drizzle over baked salmon or other fish.

STICKY PORTUGUESE

1/2 red onion, chopped

1 long red chilli, chopped

1 tsp sweet paprika

1 1/2 tsp smoked paprika

1/2 tsp coriander seed powder

2 gloves garlic, finely chopped

2 tbsp red wine vinegar

1 tbsp dry sherry or port

4 tbsp virgin olive oil

1 tsp honey or coconut syrup

1 1/2 tbsp tomato purée

1 tsp sea salt

Goes well with poultry, red meat and seafood.

homemade spice mixes

Making your own spice mixes is fun and is the best way to know exactly what's in them. Grind the seeds or use ground powders and mix in a dry bowl.

MOROCCAN

1 tsp ground coriander seeds

1 tsp ground cumin seeds

1 tsp paprika

1 tsp turmeric

1/2 tsp garlic powder

1/2 tsp onion powder

1/2 tsp black pepper

1/2 tsp sea salt

Use for tagines and stews, or to rub chicken, beef, goat or fish.

INDIAN

2 tsp sweet paprika

1 tsp ground cumin seeds

1/2 tsp ground coriander seeds

1/2 tsp ground cloves

1/2 tsp ground cinnamon

1/2 tsp ground cardamom

1/2 tsp chilli powder

1 tsp turmeric powder

1 tsp onion powder

Great for grilled meats and seafood, or a spice base for a curry. Mix with tomatoes and stock or with some coconut milk for a Sri Lankan curry.

MEXICAN FIESTA

1 tsp sweet paprika

1 tsp ground coriander seeds

1 tsp ground cumin seeds

1/2 tsp chilli powder

1/2 tsp black pepper

1/2 tsp sea salt

1 tsp dried oregano

Did someone say tacos?

SZECHUAN SALT MIX

2 tbsp sea salt

1 tbsp Szechuan peppercorn

1 tsp onion powder

1/2 tsp garlic powder

1/2 tsp chilli flakes

Sprinkle on top of grilled duck or quail, over grilled prawns or steak.

CAJUN

2 tsp paprika

2 tsp cayenne pepper

2 tsp garlic powder

2 tsp onion powder

1 tsp dried oregano

1 tsp dried thyme

1 tsp sea salt

2 tsp white pepper

Use for barbecue ribs and chicken, blackened fish and steaks, and in soups and sauces.

cashew raita

MAKES 250ML

90g cashews

Juice of 1 lemon

3/4 tsp tahini paste

1/2 tsp cumin powder

125ml water

1 tbsp extra-virgin olive oil

Pinch of salt

1/2 clove of garlic, finely chopped

1/2 medium cucumber, finely diced

1 tbsp chopped mint

Soak cashews in warm water with a dash of lemon or white wine vinegar for 4–6 hours. Rinse well and add to a food processor with all other ingredients except for cucumber and mint. Process until smooth, for about for 3–4 minutes. Remove to a small bowl and mix with finely diced cucumber and fresh mint.

hot caraway mustard

Mustard is very easy to make and there are many variations depending on the colour of the mustard seeds, the temperature of the water you use to mix the mustard and other spices and herbs you decide to add. This mustard is quite spicy but you can use warm water when mixing to make it more mild.

MAKES 250ML

3 tbsp yellow mustard seeds

1/2 tsp caraway seeds

1/2 black peppercorns

30g white mustard powder

1/2 tsp turmeric

1 tsp sea salt

2 1/2 tbsp white wine vinegar

125ml warm water (cold if you like it very hot and spicy)

Using a mortar and pestle or a food processor, grind whole mustard seeds, caraway seeds and peppercorns until partially broken but some of the seeds are still intact. Transfer to a ceramic bowl and add mustard powder, turmeric (for gorgeous bright colour), salt, vinegar and water. Mix well and transfer to a glass jar or leave covered in the bowl. Leave in the fridge for 12 hours to develop. It will keep for up to four weeks in the fridge.

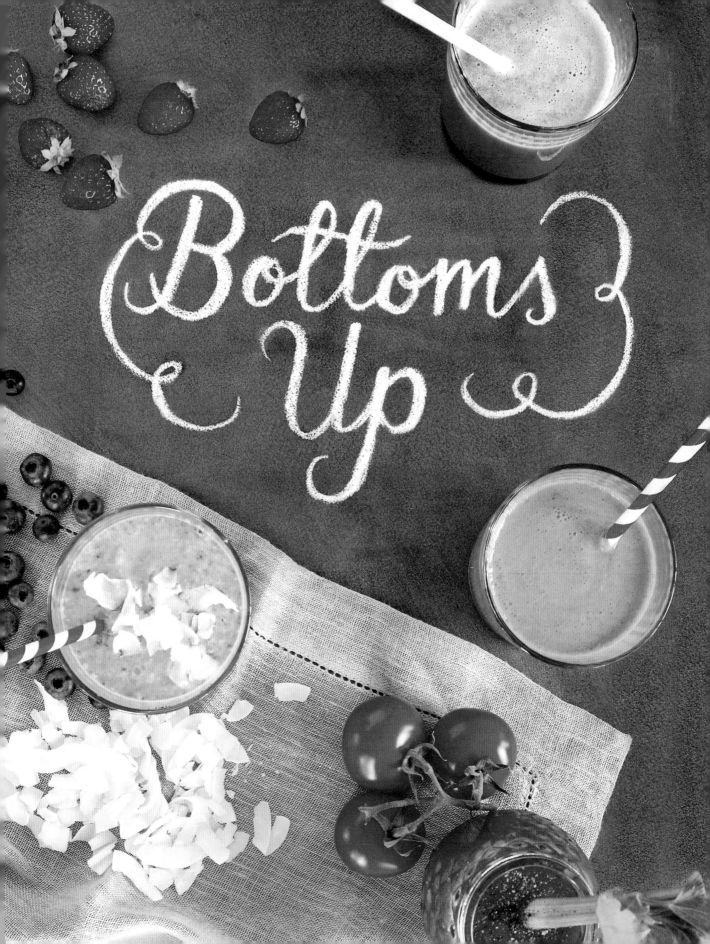

mixed berry & chocolate smoothie

This is a dessert in a glass – think black forest cake, Cherry Ripe chocolate bar or a mixed-berry chocolate pudding. It's rich in protein from whey powder and antioxidants from berries and cacao powder.

SERVES 2

160g frozen mixed berries

250ml coconut milk

2 tbsp whey protein powder

1 tsp raw cacao or cocoa powder

1 tsp sugar-free mixed berry jam

Dark chocolate shavings

Process in a blender until smooth and thick. Add a little water if using chilled coconut milk, which tends to thicken in the fridge.

aperol spritz

I fell in love with this drink in Italy, where it originates. It's made with Aperol, an aperitif similar to Campari and made with bitter orange, rhubarb, gentian and liquorice, among other ingredients. Serve as a pre-dinner drink to get your taste buds and appetite into gear. My recipe is slightly modified from the original.

SERVES 1

1 lemon slice

1 orange slice

2 tbsp orange juice

30ml Aperol

Few cubes of ice

150ml Prosecco

30ml soda water

Place lemon and orange slices on the bottom of the glass. Squeeze in orange juice and add the Aperol. Add ice and slowly pour Prosecco over. Give it a gentle stir and splash with some soda water.

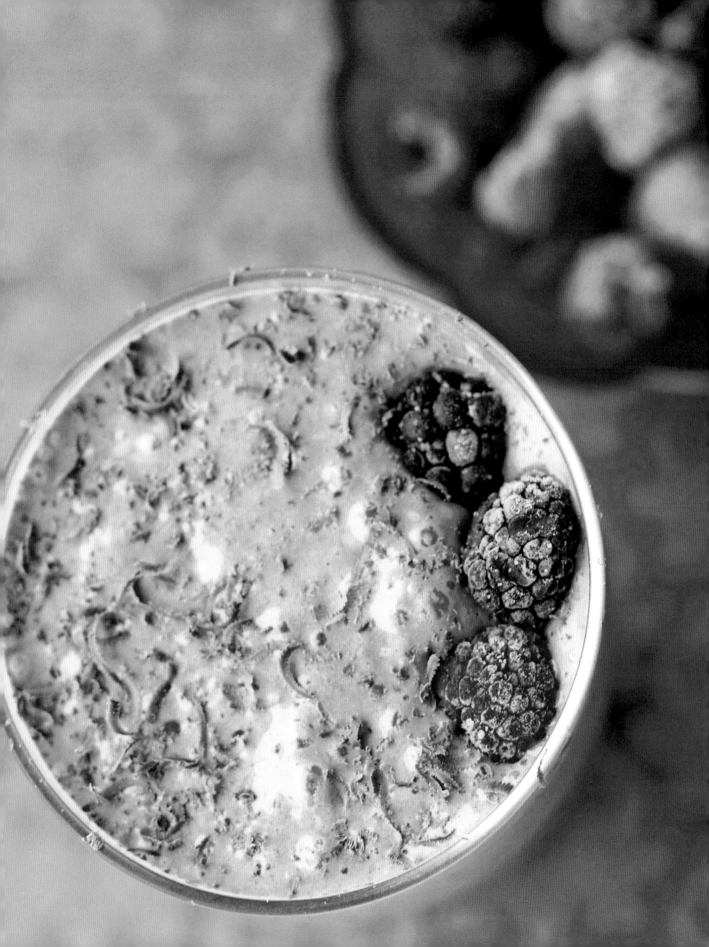

beetroot glory

This invigorating juice is a great way to start the day. Beetroot contains powerful antioxidants, lots of iron and folic acid. Paired with fragrant strawberries, crunchy green apple and carrots, this is one tasty, nutritious drink. You will need a juicer for this one.

MAKES 250–500ML

2 medium beetroots, washed

2 medium carrots, washed

3 green apples, washed and quartered

5 medium strawberries

1 celery stick

1 thumb-sized piece of fresh ginger (optional)

Ice to serve

Juice all ingredients, stir and pour over ice. Drink while fresh.

lychee lemongrass sangria

Summer weekends are not the same without a chilled jug of sangria. You might be more familiar with the red wine sangria but it's time to try something different. This white wine version is light, fragrant and slightly exotic.

MAKES ABOUT 1 LITRE

750ml white wine

1 stalk lemongrass, pale part, cut in thirds

Peel of 1 lime

1 green apple, diced

200g tinned lychees

125ml low-sugar grape juice

2 tbsp lime juice

Ice to serve

250ml soda water

Handful of fresh mint

Combine wine, lemongrass, lime peel, apple, lychees, grape juice and lime juice in a jug and refrigerate overnight. Add some ice, soda water and fresh mint when serving.

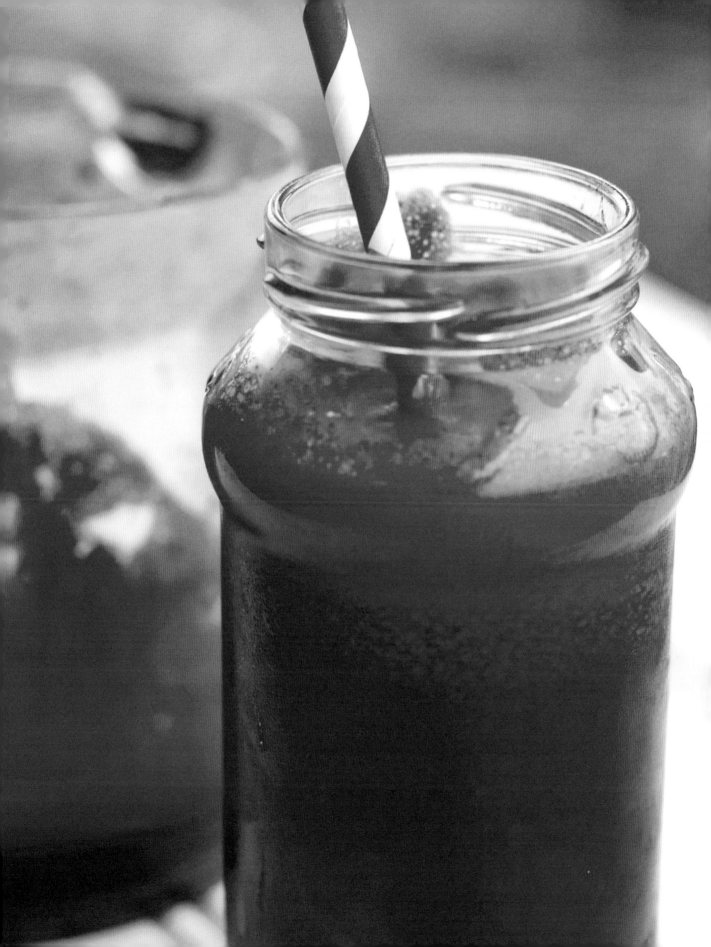

sunday bloody mary

One of my favourite drinks is a good Bloody Mary, and what makes a Bloody Mary good is the tomato juice mix you use to serve over vodka and ice. It's best and easiest to pre-mix the juice ahead of time to allow flavours and spices to fuse together. This Bloody Mary pre-mix is what I used to make during my cocktail making days.

MAKES 1 LITRE OF PRE-MIX

For the Bloody Mary pre-mix

1 litre good quality tomato juice, no added sugar

1 tbsp horseradish

Peel and juice of 1/2 orange

Peel and juice of 1/2 lemon

3 tbsp gluten-free Worcestershire sauce

1 tsp fish sauce

1/2 tsp sea salt

1/2 tsp ground black pepper

1 tbsp Tabasco or hot chilli sauce

20ml dry sherry or port

For one cocktail

Lemon wedge for rim of the glass

Sea salt for the rim of the glass

1 celery stick

50ml good quality vodka

Ice to serve

2/3 cup Bloody Mary pre-mix

1 green olive and cherry tomato

Optional: chilli celery salt

1 tsp chilli flakes

1 tsp celery seeds

1 tbsp sea salt

Combine all pre-mix ingredients in a jar or a large bottle and mix together. It can be used right away or stored in the fridge for up to three days. You can pour the mix over straight ice for a virgin Bloody Mary.

To make the cocktail, rub the rim of the glass with lemon and dip in the salt. Place the celery stick inside and pour in the vodka. Fill with ice halfway and pour the tomato pre-mix to the top. Pierce a cherry tomato and a green olive with a bamboo skewer and put in the glass to use as a stirrer.

To make chilli celery salt, grind ingredients in a mortar and pestle until well incorporated and use to dip the rim of the glass.

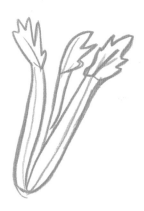

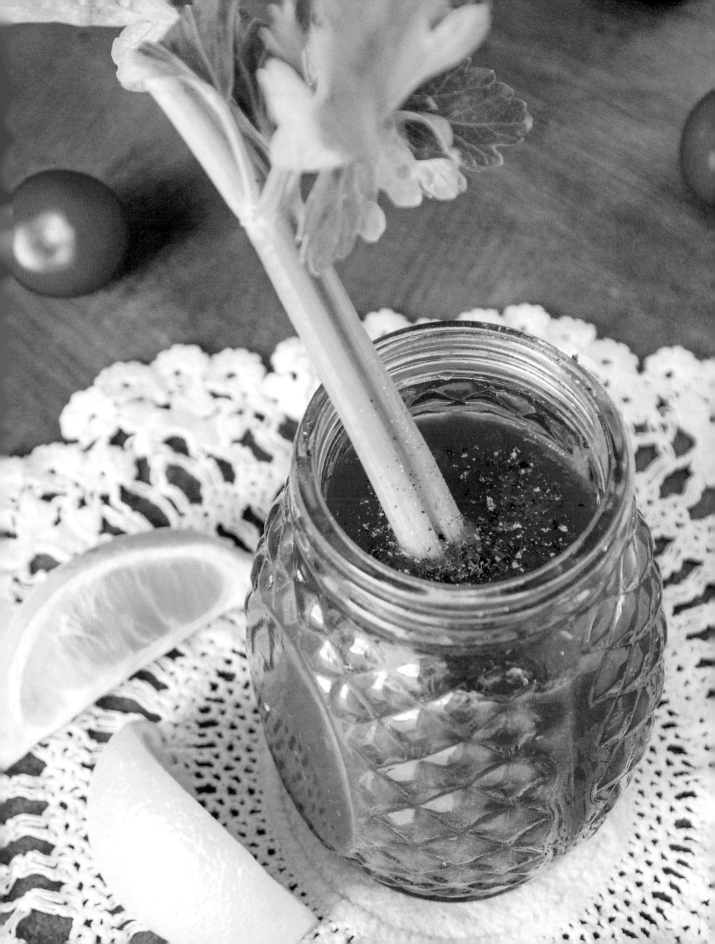

blueberry dreams

MAKES 250–375ML

100g blueberries (fresh or frozen)

75g diced mango

1 tsp vanilla extract

1 tbsp lemon juice

125ml coconut water

Ice

Combine all ingredients in a blender and purée into a smooth, thick drink. If using frozen blueberries, rinse them under hot water to thaw out quicker. Normal water or some apple juice can be used instead of coconut water.

bimka

Before I became a good cook, I was really good at making cocktails. In fact, for a little while I used to teach cocktail classes in a high-profile Sydney bar. This was one of the cocktails I made up for the menu at the time. It's named after my first dog, Bimka. I've modified it for this cookbook.

SERVES 1

20ml vodka

30ml Apple Sourz liqueur

60ml apple juice

1 tbsp fresh lime juice

5 fresh blueberries

Ice

15ml Crème de Cassis

1/2 green apple, sliced thinly

Use a mixing jug or a cocktail shaker to combine vodka, Apple Sourz, apple juice and lime juice. Drop a few blueberries on the bottom of a tall cocktail glass and fill with ice. Shake the cocktail mixture and pour over ice. Pour Crème de Cassis down the side of the glass, letting it sink to the bottom and create a gradient in the liquid. Arrange apple slices in a fan and sit on the top of the glass.

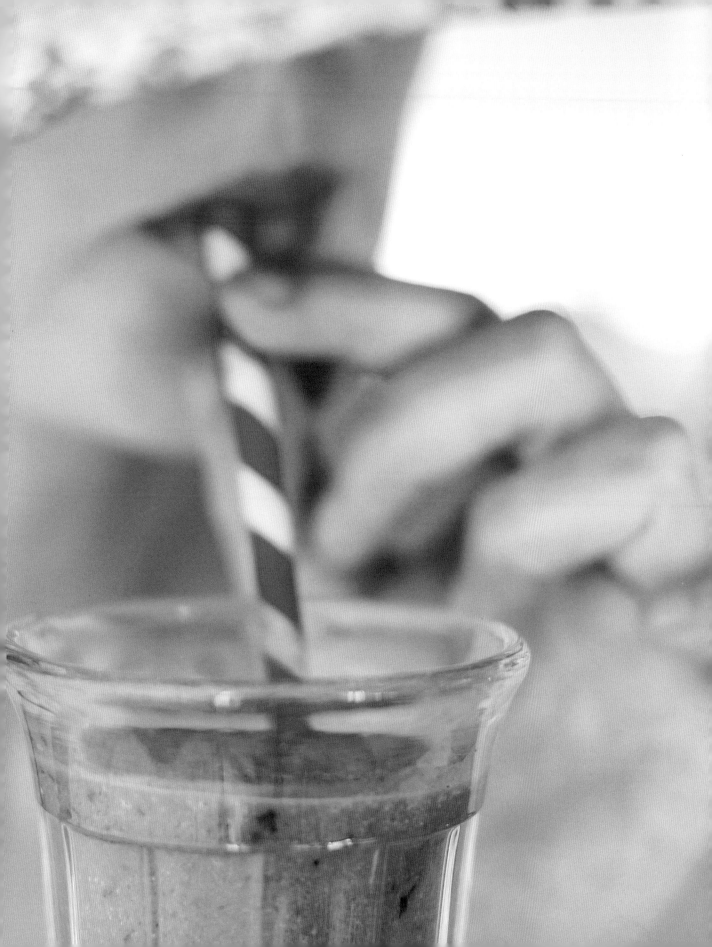

honey ginger beer

You need some dry yeast to make a homemade ginger beer as it acts as a fermenting agent and gives it that fizzy quality. Let's get one thing clear – there is bad yeast (not worth mentioning here) and then there is the beneficial kind, typically from the Saccharomyces genus, which has anti-microbial effects in the gut. Active dried yeast is absolutely paleo friendly and is used in this drink. This is a quick version that only takes 24 hours.

MAKES 1 LITRE

About a litre of boiling water

125ml raw honey

Juice and peel of 1 lemon

35g sliced fresh ginger

1 tsp dry yeast

Cool the boiled water slightly, so it's okay to touch. Combine water, honey, lemon juice and peel, ginger and yeast in a large bowl and cover loosely with muslin cloth or plastic wrap. Set aside at room temperature for 24 hours.

Skim off any scum that has risen to the top with a slotted spoon. Strain the liquid through a sieve and pour into clean glass bottles or jars (leave a little room at the top). Keep well chilled in the fridge and serve over ice with extra fresh lemon and some fresh mint.

strawberry kisses

MAKES 250–375ML

5–6 medium strawberries

165ml coconut milk

1/2 tsp vanilla extract

1 tsp almond butter

Ice

Combine all ingredients in a blender and purée into a smooth, thick drink. If using frozen strawberries, rinse them under hot water to thaw out quicker.

raspberry gin fizz

This cocktail is inspired by another drink I used to make during my cocktail days. You could use vodka instead of gin and strawberries instead of raspberries. Chambord is a French raspberry liqueur but you could use another good-quality variety.

To make raspberry purée, blend all ingredients in a blender. Store in a squeeze bottle.

In a cocktail shaker, combine gin, Chambord, raspberry purée, vanilla, lemon juice and ice. Shake well and strain as you pour over fresh ice cubes in a tumbler. Top up with soda water and garnish with fresh mint and raspberries.

SERVES 1

For the raspberry purée

65g raspberries, fresh or frozen and thawed

125ml water

1 tsp natural sweetener (e.g. raw honey)

For the cocktail

30ml good-quality gin

30ml Chambord

35g raspberry purée

1/2 tsp vanilla extract

1 tbsp lemon juice

Handful of ice

Ice cubes, to serve

125ml soda water

Fresh mint and raspberries, to serve

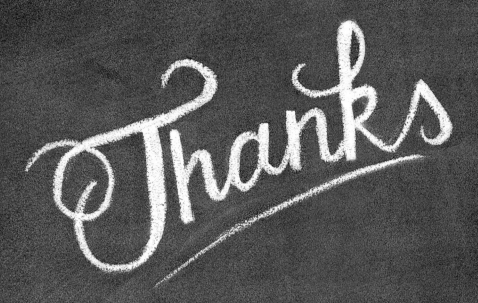

Thanks

This cookbook was made possible with the support of many friends, and strangers. Whether you were with me through the whole process or helped out on occasion by cleaning up my kitchen mess and testing my food, I want to thank you from the bottom of my heart.

Special mention to some of my close friends and loved ones who had to put up with me for the last few months.

Matti Puckridge, Carla Hackett, Jodie McLeod, Tim Lucas, Gloria Tong, Stephen Lead, Simon Wright, Lilli Altendorfer, Ursula Everett, Eric Auld, Melody Puckridge, Elle Patrikis, Danielle Szetho and my family.

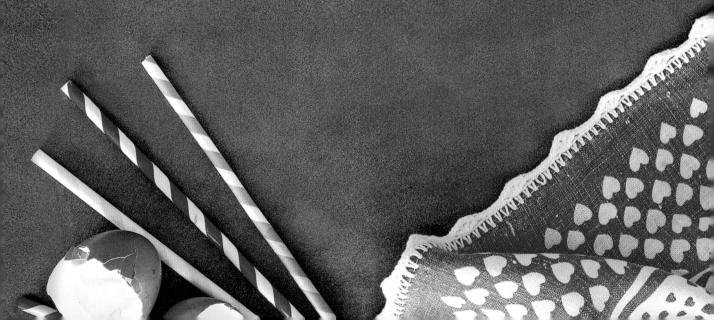

— thank you —

And a huge thank you to all my Pozible supporters:

Alison Mitchell
Andrew Wyers
Anna
Annalea Johnston
Annette Boehm
Ben Askins
Ben Webster
Bruno Mattarollo
Cameron Barrie
Caroline Strudwick-Brown
Cate Prentice
Chris Stephens
Cyrus Eftos
Danielle Szetho
Deb Davidson
Deborah Caddy
Dmitry Baranovskiy
Enrique Salceda
Evan Ford
Freya Davidson
Garmisch & Tim Riley
Gemma Starzec
Gloria Tong
Hayli Chwang
Inna Yankevych
Jacquie Collins
Jared Wyles
Jason Crane
Jennifer Manefield
Josh Ruscheinsky

Jodi Morgan
John Rimmer
Julie Keith
Justin Koke
Justin Vön Ong
Kath Hamilton
Kerensa Anderson
Kris Owen
Kristian Milos
Kristina Ljubicic
Kurumi Honda
Lauren Whitehead
Leanne Barry
Lexi Thorn
Lily Perthuis
Lisa Miller
Luisa Bolzic
Magi Hernandez
Marcus Stenbeck
Marinka Bil
Mark Cowley
Matt Willis
Maxine Sherrin
Michael Koukoullis
Mychelle Vanderburg
Nadine Richter
Narelle Hickling-Thompson
Nathan de Vries
Nicole Smith

Patrick Cranshaw
Pauline Allen
Petter Lundmark
Rashelle Zelaznik
Rebecca Axon
Rod Tobin
Ryan Junee
Ryan Kitching
Sanna Lundmark
Shari Henderson
Sharon Worster
Simon Ratner
Simon Wright
Sophia Molodysky
Sophie Wright
Srini Madhavan
Stephen Cox
Stephen Mason-Ellen
Steve Gilles
Sue Cotterell
Sugendran Ganess
Tim Lucas
Toby Forage
Tony Hall
Trent Brown
Ursula Everett
And Niulife for yummy coconut goodies

references

BOOKS

Enig, Mary and Fallon, Sally. *Eat Fat, Lose Fat: The Healthy Alternative to Trans Fats.* New York: Plume, 2006.

Fallon, Sally. *Nourishing Traditions: The Cookbook That Challenges Politically Correct Nutrition and the Diet Dictocrats.* Lanham: New Trends Publishing Inc, US, 2003.

Jaminet, P and Jaminet, S-C. *Perfect Health Diet: Four Steps To Renewed Health, Youthful Vitality, and Long Life.* YingYang Press, 2010.

Sanfillipp, Diane. *Practical Paleo: A Customised Approach to Health and a Whole-foods Lifestyle.* Las Vegas: Victory Belt Publishing, 2012.

Wolf, Robb. *The Paleo Solution: The Original Human Diet.* Las Vegas: Victory Belt Publishing, 2010.

ONLINE RESOURCES

Ballantyne, S 2012, *The Science and Art of Paleofying—Part 1 Paleo Flours*, accessed 17 March, 2013

Ballantune, S 2012, *The Autoimmune Protocol,* accessed 18 March, 2013

Byrnes, S 2002, *Myths of Vegetarianism,* accessed 20 March, 2013

Carrera-Bastos P, Fontes Villalba M, O'Keefe JH, Lindeberg S, Cordain L, 2011, *The Western Diet and Lifestyle and Diseases of Civilization*, PDF, accessed 24 March, 2013

Crawford, A 2013, *Activating Nuts and Seeds,* accessed 19 March 2013

Eades, M.R 2009, *Nutrition and health in agriculturalists and hunter-gatherers,* accessed 15 December, 2012

Eaton SB, Cordain L, Sparling PB, Cantwell JD., 2009, *Evolution, Body Composition and Insulin Resistance*, PDF, accessed 24 March, 2013

Johnson, K 2013, *Health Benefits of Bone Broth,* accessed 3 March, 2013

Kresser, C 2012, *Shaking up The Salt Myth: When Salt Reduction May Be Warranted,* accessed 15 December, 2012

Kresser, C 2013, *Does Red Meat Cause Inflammation?,* accessed 15 April, 2013

Kresser, C 2013, *Red Meat: It Does a Body Good,* accessed 23 March, 2012

Lindeberg, S, Jönsson, T, Granfeldt, Y, Borgstrand, E, Soffman, J, Sjöström, K, and Ahrén, B 2007, *A Palaeolithic diet improves glucose tolerance more than a Mediterranean-like diet in individuals with ischaemic heart disease,* accessed 17 March, 2013

Taylor, J n.d., *Paleo Diet Carbohydrate List and Carb Counter,* accessed 18 March, 2013

Satin, M 2012, *Salt and Our Health,* accessed 16 March, 2013

Sisson, M 2009, *The Primal Blueprint Carbohydrate Curve,* accessed 19 March, 2013

Wolf, Robb. 2013, *What is the Paleo Diet?,* accessed 20 January, 2013

Myths & Truths About Nutrition, 2000, accessed 18 March, 2013

It's the Beef, 2000, accessed 13 February, 2013

GRAINS & LEGUMES

Freed, D.L.J 1999, *Do Dietary Lectins Cause Disease?*, accessed 15 March, 2013

Jaminet, P 2010, *Wheat Is a Cause of Many Diseases, I: Leaky Gut*, accessed 16 March, 2013

Jaminet, P 2011, *Why We Get Fat: Food Toxins*, accessed 16 March, 2013

Kresser, C 2011, *9 Steps To Perfect Health #1: Don't Eat Toxins*, accessed 19 December, 2013

Rose, A 2013, *Phytic Acid*, accessed 17 March, 2013

Sgourakis, E 2012, *Don't Go Nuts*, accessed 19 March, 2013

Less Bad but Not Good: Pseudograins and Non-gluten Grains n.d., accessed 17 March, 2013

Soy Alert n.d., accessed 10 March, 2013

SUGAR/SWEETENERS

Appleton, N and Jacobs, GN 2010, *141 Reasons Sugar Ruins Your Health*, accessed 21 March, 2013

Cordain, L, n.d., *Sugar Content of Fruit*, accessed March 22, 2013

Fallon Morell, S and Nagel R 2009, *Agave Nectar: Worse Than We Thought*, accessed 23 March, 2013

Kresser, C 2012, *Ask Chris: Is Fructose Really That Bad?*, accessed 29 February, 2013

Sanfilippo, D, n.d., *Guide to Sweeteners*, PDF, accessed 22 March, 2013

Sisson, M 2010, *The Definitive Guide to Sugar*, accessed 21 March, 2013

Sisson, M 2011, *A Primal Primer: Stevia*, accessed 23 March, 2013

FATS & OILS

Champ, CE 2012, *Checking Your Oil: The Definitive Guide to Cooking with Fat*, accessed 22 March, 2013

Cordain, L, n.d., *Fats and Fatty Acids*, accessed 22 March, 2013

Masterjohn, C 2012, *Good Fats, Bad Fats: Separating Facts from Fiction*, accessed 22 March, 2013

Rose, L 2011, *The Complete Guide to Fats and Oils – What to Cook With (or not), What to Avoid and Why*, accessed 24 March, 2013

Taylor, J 2010, *Omega 6 and 3 in Nuts, Oils, Meat and Fish. Tools to Get It Right*, accessed 19 March, 2013

Sanfilippo, D, n.d., *Guide to Fats & Oils*, PDF, accessed March 24 2012

Sisson, M 2008, *The Definitive Guide to Cholesterol*, accessed 22 March, 2013

Myths and Truths About Cholesterol, 2009, accessed 23 March, 2013

What's Cooking America n.d., Type of Cooking Fats and Oils – Smoking Points of Fats and Oils, accessed 22 March, 2013

DAIRY

Kresser, C 2013, *For A Healthy Heart, Stick to Butter*, accessed 24 March, 2013

Kresser, C 2011, *Dairy: Foods of The Gods or Neolithic Agent of Disease?*, accessed 24 March, 2013

Kubal, Amy 2012, *Seven Shades of Paleo*, accessed 24 March, 2013

Sisson, M 2009, *Is All Cheese Created Equal?*, accessed 24 March, 2013

Sisson, M 2010, *The Definitive Guide to Dairy*, accessed 24 March, 2013

recipe index

notes

—————————— notes ——————————